# ACUPUNCTURE
## and
# MOXIBUSTION

# ACUPUNCTURE
# and
# MOXIBUSTION

## A Handbook for the
## Barefoot Doctors of China

TRANSLATED BY Martin Elliot Silverstein,
I-Lok Chang, and
Nathaniel Macon

SCHOCKEN BOOKS / NEW YORK

First published by SCHOCKEN BOOKS 1975
Copyright © 1975 by Schocken Books Inc.

*Library of Congress Cataloging in Publication Data*

Hopei, China (Province). Wei sheng t'ing.
    Acupuncture and moxibustion.

    Translation of Chen chiu.
    Includes indexes.
    1. Acupuncture. I. Silverstein, Martin Elliot.
II. Chang, I-Lok. III. Macon, Nathaniel, 1926-
IV. Title. [DNLM: 1. Acupuncture. 2. Moxibustion.
WB369 H791c]
RM184.H625 1975        615'.892        74-26919

# A Disclaimer

The translators of this volume are just that—translators. We have attempted, by combining our skills, to produce a valid English-language version of a Mainland Chinese manual for rural paramedical technicians, known picturesquely as "barefoot doctors." The nature of the subject, the need for medical interpretation of Chinese descriptions of symptoms and diseases, and the peculiar topology of the designated anatomical meridians have forced us at times to considerable interpretation. An earlier transliteration was perhaps more free of translator's subjectivity, but lacked reasonable coherence.

We emphasize that we are not, and never have been, experts on or practitioners of acupuncture, moxibustion, or any of the Chinese medical arts. We do not know whether these procedures are, indeed, valid therapeutic techniques. We have not been in contact with the authors or publishers of the original Chinese work, feeling that this separation helped to preserve the freshness of our viewpoint and the integrity of our translation. The translation is not authorized by either the Chinese or the United States government.

We present this translation to the English-language reader without advocacy, evaluation, or recommendation. We believe that, as an attempt by the Chinese government to bring order out of a chaotic field for its own practitioners, it deserves a special place in the acupuncture literature. As an item of medical curiosa and historical interest, it stands on its merits. To the layman interested in acupuncture, we offer it as the clearest, simplest description we have been able to find in the Chinese literature. To the Western physician, we offer it as a reasonable starting point in his investigations of a much-discussed and potentially valuable tool in his efforts to treat human ills.

# Acknowledgments

The translators are deeply indebted to Mr. Roy Andres, who, during his visit to China to establish telecommunications for President Nixon's visit there, procured for us a copy of this handbook. We also wish to acknowledge the valuable help of Miss Lynda Sun, Dr. Mabelle Cremer, and Susan and Patricia Macon.

# Preface

The Cultural Revolution has reached an extremely favorable phase. The vast revolutionary masses of the country are striving to realize the new goals of our great leader, Chairman Mao—striving for total victory in the Cultural Revolution of the proletariat. The proletariat group of the medical world is most actively responding to the great call of Chairman Mao—to bring emphasis on medical activities into the farming villages. Thus, a great revolutionary zeal is generated among medical workers to live in the farming villages and to serve the peasants of China.

As we are determined to follow the new direction Chairman Mao set for medical workers, we have produced this volume. Its aim is to meet the urgent need of the medical workers who serve the farming community. To meet this pressing need we have selected and compiled information from past publications on basic medical topics of interest to farm-community practitioners. These materials antedate the Cultural Revolution of the proletariat. Despite the great interest of Chairman Mao, there are still inadequacies in that these sources are written for the urban medical worker; the level is different and departs from the practical need of the farming villages. Because of the urgent need for these source materials, we are unable to prepare a complete revision appropriate for the purposes of the farm medical worker. Therefore, we sincerely hope that the vast number of workers who will use this text will, as a result of the problems arising from practical experience, supply us with a strenuous critique and communicate their suggestions for improving the book.

The People's Health Press
March 1968
Address correspondence to:
Editor's Office
People's Health Press
15 Ing Tse Street
Chung Wun District
Peking

# Thoughts of Chairman Mao

The spirit of Comrade Doctor Pai Chieu-en is characterized by his selflessness and concern for other people, as shown by his high sense of responsibility and his great love for the masses. Every Communist Party member must learn from his life.

*In Memory of Pai Chieu-en,* December 21, 1939

We are the army for liberation of the people; we have only one purpose—to serve the people. . . . Because our sole aim is the service of the people, we invite criticism of our shortcomings by any man. Providing the criticism is correct, we will correct our shortcomings.

*In the Service of the People,* September 8, 1944

The peasant is the main concern of this phase of the Chinese cultural movement. Abolishment of illiteracy, universal education, the People's Culture, the People's Health—are they not empty phrases if we leave out the 360 million peasants?

*A Treatise on Unified Government,* April 24, 1945

We will unify the ancient and the modern; we will combine Chinese and Western medicine. We will form a solid uniform battlefront (line) so as to strive and work for the health and well-being of a great people.

Theme of the 1950 National Medical Conference

We must energetically strive to prevent and treat disease among our people, constantly expanding the scope of medical work available to the people.

*A Treatise on Unified Government,* April 24, 1945

# Author's Preface

To meet the present need to provide medical training to the farming communities through the agency of field paramedics, I have organized a group to edit the present text on acupuncture and moxibustion. The content of the text emphasizes the basic techniques and the special characteristics of the subject, giving special attention to the needs of agricultural communities.

The text is divided into two major parts. The first part introduces basic aspects of the techniques and several basic methods of actual physical application, along with a discussion on ninety-two commonly used anatomical acupuncture points. The second part deals with the therapy for certain common illnesses, including forty-nine diseases commonly occurring in farming communities. The therapy for each disease is introduced with an evaluation of its effectiveness. The fewest number of body points necessary for the treatment are indicated. Practicability is stressed so that a beginner can master the subject and apply it without much difficulty.

The preparation of a text in this field is a new experiment to us. In order to be certain that the text will accommodate the actual need of the farming community, we have given the first draft to the students in medical workers' training classes, organized discussion groups afterward, and requested the comment of the instructors. We have made several revisions, and finally arrived at the present text. We realize that, because of the physical differences between localities and the differences in the educational levels of the readers, the content of the instruction may have to be amplified or simplified to suit the setting and the demands of the community.

The need for more medical experience in this subject and the lack of time for editing have no doubt resulted in many shortcomings and errors in the text. We sincerely hope that the instructors and the readers, through their practical use of the text, will communicate to us suggestions for future editions.

We must mention also that we are preparing a text entitled *The Essentials of Chinese Medical Methods*. Together with the present text, the two texts may be used for a one-year training course on an apprentice basis.

The Department of Health, Ho Pei Province

November 1965

# A Handbook on Acupuncture Medicine

---

Preliminary Edition (61,000 Chinese characters)

Prepared by the Health Department of Ho Pei Province

Published by People's Health Press

Peking's Publications Permit No. 46

15 Ing Tse Street, Chung Wun District, Peking

Printed by the second Shing Hua printing office

Distributed by Peking's Shing Hua distributor, available at all Shing Hua bookstores

Unified Book No. 14048.3179

Price 0.17 yen

First Edition—1st printing, December 1965

First Edition—8th printing, January 1970

Number printed: 813,101—1,793,100

# Contents

---

PART ONE
## Fundamentals of
## Acupuncture and Moxibustion

# Fundamentals of Acupuncture and Moxibustion

# Section I:

## Treatment by Acupuncture and Moxibustion

Acupuncture and moxibustion are two methods of treatment that have their origins in prehistoric China. Specifically, the therapeutic technique of acupuncture is accomplished by inserting slim metal needles into specified points on the skin of the human body. Moxibustion is a closely related therapeutic technique in which heat is applied to the acupoints by igniting products made from the dried leaves of the moxa plant (wormwood: *Artemisia moxa*). The techniques are related in that both the acupuncture needles and the moxibustion heat are applied to the same system of anatomical points on the skin. In many cases the techniques are used in conjunction with each other, and therefore they are commonly discussed in the same context.

# Section II:

## The Advantages of Acupuncture and Moxibustion Therapy

For several thousand years acupuncture and moxibustion have been a favorite of the Great Proletariat. Some of the reasons for this are:

### 1. Simplicity, Economy, and Availability

The only materials required are slim metal needles, moxa wicks, alcohol, and absorbent cotton. With these you can administer treatment any time and at any place. The equipment is easy to set up and convenient to use, and the need for the patients to buy medicine is greatly reduced. The materials are inexpensive to manufacture and purchase. Consequently, the cost of treatment is minimal.

## 2. Easily Learned and Applied Techniques

Acupuncture medicine requires:

a. Diagnosis of the patient's illness in acupuncture terms
b. Knowledge of anatomical positions of treatment spots
c. Knowing the combination of spots that results in the cure of the diagnosed ailment
d. Knowing the methods of inserting, manipulating, and extracting the needle, and dexterity in doing so

## 3. Wide Therapeutic Applications

Acupuncture has been used successfully in diseases of the classic categories of internal medicine, pediatrics, dermatology, obstetrics, and gynecology, and in lieu of surgery.

## 4. Safety and Reliability

One need only pay strictest attention to following technique instructions and to skin sterilization to insure that no dangerous or unreliable consequences will occur.

# Section III:
## The Technique
## of Acupuncture

### 1. Description and Classification of the Basic Acupuncture Instruments

Though there are several varieties of needles, the two types most commonly used are the slim needle *(hao chen)* and the trocar-tipped needle *(san-lin chen)*.[1] The hao is more widely used, tends to be slimmer, and comes in several lengths including 0.5 chun, 1.0 chun, 1.5 chuns, 2.0 chuns, 3.0 chuns, 5.0 chuns, etc.[2] There are four commonly used calibers or gauges, which are designated as 26, 28, 30, and 32. The slim hao is used for treating ailments. The usually shorter, sharp-tipped san-lin has a thicker caliber, and often is used in letting blood and for other incisions.

## 2. Finger Strength Development and Needle Rotation Practice

The first step for the beginner is developing finger strength by practice and achieving dexterity in rotation. These should be accomplished before acupuncture is attempted on a patient.

a. How to develop finger strength: Fold each of twenty sheets of single-ply tissue paper in fours so as to make a thick, resilient pad. Tie the pad firmly with strong thread. Hold the pad with the left hand. Using the thumb, index, and middle fingers of the right hand to hold the needle point against the paper pad, insert the needle, while rotating it clockwise and counterclockwise. Begin using a 0.5 chun hao needle (1.6 cm. round needle). Then proceed to practice successively with the 1.0 chun (3.2 cm.), 2.0 chuns (6.4 cm.), and 3.0 chuns (9.6 cm.) hao needles. Continue practicing until you can accomplish rotation-insertion easily and without force. When you can do this easily you will find that you are able, quickly and skillfully, to accomplish rotation-insertion into the human skin (Fig. 1).

b. How to practice needle motions within the body: Roll some cotton into a ball and tightly wrap standard cotton string around it, about ten times. Hold the wrapped cotton ball in the left hand and the acupuncture needle in the right hand between the thumb, index, and middle fingers. Insert the needle into the wrapped ball and rotate the needle clockwise and counterclockwise. Then try to ac-

1. The principal distinction between these two types is that the former has a circular cross section and the tip has no cutting edges, tapering evenly to a point, while the latter has a similar body with a tip cut to a triangular cross section reducing to a needle-sharp point. The hao is comparable to a surgical noncutting needle; the san-lin resembles a surgical cutting needle.—Trans.
2. One Chinese chun is equivalent to approximately 3.2 cm.—Trans.

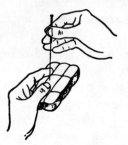 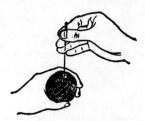

**Fig. 1** Finger strength exercise (a)    **Fig. 2** Finger strength exercise (b)

company this with a gentle inward and outward motion (deep to superficial, and vice versa). After you have practiced this for a while, make the ball larger by once again wrapping it with ten wraps of cotton string and try it again. You should practice every day, increasing the thickness of your cotton ball every day in the same way, until you have no difficulty in the simultaneous rotation and reciprocal motion of the needle. Your skill will improve as the ball grows, and you will be ready to perform the motion on the human body (Fig. 2).

### 3. Special Precautions

a. Make sure that your needle is not bent or rusty, and that the point is sharp. If the needle is not in good condition, replace it. If you do not replace it you risk problems on inserting and extracting, and even breaking the needle.

b. Be sure to sterilize each needle by boiling it in water for no less than ten minutes or soaking it in warm 75 per cent [sic] alcohol for fifteen minutes.

c. Before inserting an acupuncture needle, select the relevant spot precisely and decide how deep the needle should be inserted. The size of the patient—depending upon how fat or thin he is—will influence the choice of needle length.

d. Position the patient so that the relevant spot can be reached

6

easily, and so that the patient can rest comfortably in that position for a long time. Tell the patient not to move while you are inserting the needle. Some suggested positions include having the patient supine when you operate on acupuncture points on the face, abdomen, arms, and legs. To approach the back and the back of the leg, the patient should be prone. To reach the hip joint, the patient should be positioned on the opposite side. It is convenient to have the patient sitting in a chair with a headrest when you insert needles into the head and into the extremities.

e. After you have selected proper anatomical points for insertion, mark the spots with imaginary crosses using your fingertips.

f. The acupuncturist's hands should be washed clean with soap and water before every treatment. Then use 75 per cent [sic] alcohol on absorbent cotton to clean the fingers for two or three minutes just prior to the insertion. The patient's skin at the anatomical site to be punctured should be cleansed in the same way, using a cotton ball soaked in alcohol. The skin should be cleansed in concentric circles from the center outward to achieve antisepsis.

g. Reassure patients who are having treatment for the first time. Explain that the treatment is not very painful. It is important that the patient not be frightened so that he will not faint and fall during treatment. Be sure that weak patients or patients who have a history of fainting are lying down. If during the procedure the patient begins to feel dizzy, see stars, or perspire excessively and complain of nausea, stop the procedure immediately and administer the resuscitative treatment described in the later section on neurogenic shock.

h. The depth of needle insertion discussed in later chapters is intended for the treatment of adults. Acupuncture in children requires precaution. Insertion is made to much shallower depths, usually two or three tenths of a chun (0.6 to 1.0 cm.). It is extremely important that children not be allowed to move about during treatment. Movement increases the difficulty of insertion and needle manipulation.

i. *Certain anatomical points must be avoided in pregnant women:*

It is absolutely forbidden to puncture certain points during pregnancy. In addition, it is preferable in that condition to avoid punctures in fingers and toes (such as 1.4, 2.1, 9.4, 4.1, and 3.11).

### 4. Determination of the Angle between Needle and Skin Prior to Insertion

The angle will be affected by the anatomical site of the acupuncture point and by the condition of the patient and the seriousness of the illness. In general, there are three positions for the needle: (a) perpendicular to the skin, (b) at a 45-degree angle to the skin, and (c) almost parallel to the skin (Fig. 3).

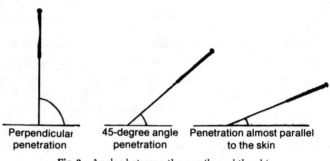

| Perpendicular penetration | 45-degree angle penetration | Penetration almost parallel to the skin |

**Fig. 3**  Angles between the needle and the skin

a. Perpendicular to the skin: This is the method most often used. It is particularly suitable for points over heavy tissue.

b. The 45-degree insertion: This method is used at anatomical sites over thin musculature and over anatomical structures that are easily injured. Such areas occur, for example, on the head, face, and breast.

c. Parallel to or at a very acute angle to the skin (sometimes called skin contour insertion): This method is used principally for certain areas on the head and face, and over some of the vital organs.

### 5. Technique of Inserting the Needle

Three methods are commonly used:

a. Rotation-insertion: This is the most common method. It is usually used with the noncutting hao needle. The right hand holds the body of the needle, with the point of the needle aimed directly at the curative point, touching the skin lightly. Now with slight pressure pierce the outer skin, and then slowly rotate the needle while inserting deeper and deeper. Success with this method depends on proper guidance with the left hand. There are three different methods of guiding with your left hand:

i. *Single-finger pressure:* Holding the needle with the right hand, the left thumb is placed close to the curative point and downward pressure is exerted by this left thumb. The needle is then placed against the skin close to the nail of the left thumb and rotated as it is inserted downward. This method is suitable for the insertion of short needles, for example at points 2.2 and 1.2 (Fig. 4).

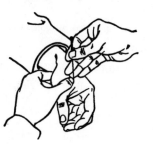
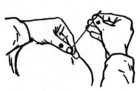

**Fig. 4**  Single-finger press        **Fig. 5**  Two-finger press

ii. *Two-finger pressure:* The body or stem of the needle is held in the right hand between the thumb, index, and middle fingers. Seize the needle just above the tip with the left thumb and index finger and so place the point of the needle at the curative spot on the skin. With quick downward pressure exerted by the left thumb and index finger, the needle point is inserted into the skin at the curative point. Simultaneously, the fingers of the right hand are used to exert downward pressure and to rotate. This method is suitable for the management of long needles such as those used at 11.3 and 3.7 (Fig. 5).

iii. *The pinch method:* When the dermis is thin or loose, the skin at the curative point may be pinched and tented between the left thumb and forefinger so that the curative point presents at the top of the pyramid of skin. Such points occur on the face at 15.1, 14.11, etc. The right hand is used as previously described to insert and rotate the needle into the curative point (Fig. 6).

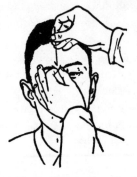

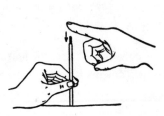

**Fig. 6** The pinch method      **Fig. 7** Needle guide tube

b. Stabbing: The trocar-pointed san-lin needle held in the right hand is stabbed through the skin at the curative point to a depth of 0.2 to 0.3 chun (0.6 to 1.0 cm.). The left hand is used to stabilize the skin at the point of entry.

c. Using a tube to guide the needle: A rather long hao needle is inserted through the lumen of a glass tube. The bottom of the tube and the needle point are pressed against the curative point, using the left hand to guide the tube and the right forefinger to tap the head of the needle rapidly, causing it to pierce the skin. The guide is then removed and the needle is inserted to the desired depth by the rotation-insertion method (Fig. 7). This method is particularly useful when treating children and adults who are afraid of pain.

### 6. The Patient's Sensations during Acupuncture

When the needle is inserted at the correct point to the correct depth, the patient often complains of aching, a numb and heavy feeling, and a sensation of pressure at that point. At the same time the acupuncturist senses a gripping and tugging of the needle. If he does not feel this pulling and tugging sensation through the needle, he may try to obtain it by moderately raising and lowering the needle while continuing the rotation. After the tugging is sensed, the acupuncturist's subsequent maneuvers will depend on the patient's condition.[3] In the case of some patients or some anatomical acupuncture points, Ch'i may not be sensed. When this happens it is wise to leave the needle in the skin for some time; the desired curative effect will be obtained.

You should not expect the same response in every acupuncture treatment. The skill and knowledge of the therapist, the anatomical point, the depth of insertion, the degree and direction of rotation, the angle of insertion, the speed of push-pull, and the patient's emotional and physical state and body build will affect both the patient's response and the acupuncturist's observations relative to this response. These responses may vary both in intensity and in the degree of extension from the puncture site. Good results require skill and sensitivity on the part of the acupuncturist.

### 7. Increasing and Decreasing Ch'i Energy by Hand Manipulation

Hand manipulations of the already inserted needle serve to increase Ch'i (to tone) and to release Ch'i (to tap). The choice of method depends on the patient's general condition and on the nature of the diagnosis. In terms of Chinese medicine, if the patient is feeble, toning is usually indicated; if the patient is physically strong, tapping is the choice. If the disease is feverous, has pronounced symptoms, and is acute, tap; if it is nonfeverous, has vague symptoms, is chronic, use toning. For those classes of diseases that are both "hot" and "cold," or which are observed to be both "concrete" and "amorphous," use the half-and-half method, which is one of the three types we are about to describe.

There are many hand manipulations for toning and tapping. The three most commonly used techniques are:

a. Push-pull method: This is begun after insertion is complete and

3. On occasion, when the acupuncturist becomes aware that he has located the node and found Ch'i, he whispers, *"Te Ch'i!"*

Ch'i has been felt. In order to tone, insert the needle to a shallower depth and then proceed to a deeper depth. Return the needle upward without quite bringing it to its original depth and then push it somewhat deeper, using greater force on the downstroke than on the upstroke. Repeat this push-pull until by increments you reach the desired depth. In order to tap, insert the needle to the maximum desired depth and then raise it to a somewhat shallower level. Using greater force on the upstroke than on the downstroke, repeat this push-pull process until by decrements you have reached the desired shallow level.

b. Rotation method: This is begun after the needle is inserted to the correct depth and Ch'i has been struck. To tone, rotate the needle clockwise by moving the thumb forward. Return the thumb and needle partway, and begin the clockwise motion again. Place emphasis on the forward motion of the thumb.[4] To tap, place the emphasis on the counterclockwise motion of the needle, that is, the backward motion of the thumb (Fig. 8).

### Rotation method

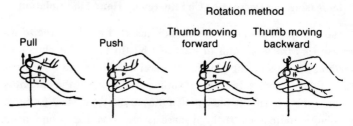

| Pull | Push | Thumb moving forward | Thumb moving backward |

**Fig. 8**   Push-pull method and rotation method

c. Equal toning and tapping method: After inserting the needle point and finding Ch'i, the acupuncturist rotates the needle between the thumb and index finger evenly in clockwise and counterclockwise directions. Alternatively, the needle may be lifted up and down

4. A later manual entitled *Acupuncture Anaesthesia Handbook,* published in 1972 by the Canton People's Liberation Hospital (Unified Publication No. 14111.95), indicates that the rate of rotation is two or three times per second. It suggests that the clockwise rotation is through an angle between 180 and 360 degrees. The counterclockwise return is between 90 and 180 degrees.—Trans.

with equal strength. This is one of the most common bedside methods.

Often, using any one of these three types of methods, the needle is not extracted right away. Instead, it is left in place for a specified time. This process is called the *liu chen,* which means leaving the needle in place. Its purpose is to enhance the toning or tapping previously attained. It is not a method of toning or tapping in itself.

These methods should not be used by rote. The choice should be determined by the clinical condition of the patient. For example, in children and weak patients the treatment should be diminished; patients who are nonresponsive or who are of strong body but seriously ill should take a heavier treatment.

### 8. Extracting the Needle

After the process of inserting and manipulating and the passive phase, the needle must be removed. To remove the needle, take a sterile cotton ball in the left hand and press on the skin at the point of entry. With the right hand rotate the needle very gently and remove it slowly and smoothly. The removal must not be performed abruptly. After extracting the needle, immediately place the cotton ball over the needle hole and press gently a few times over this point of entry to prevent bleeding.

### 9. What to Do when There Is Difficulty in Removing the Needle

Usually it is not difficult to remove the acupuncture needle. However, if during the passive phase the patient should move, the needle may be bent. It is difficult to remove a bent needle without risking danger to the patient's tissues. When the needle is bent, the acupuncturist cannot rotate the needle or pull it out without this risk. As a first step he should return the patient to the original therapeutic position. The curve of the bent needle should be carefully ascertained. Then, using the right hand to steady the needle, utilize the left thumb and left index finger to press the skin back down and around the curve of the needle. When the bend of the

13

needle is reached, slowly extract the needle by using a gentle push-pull motion. Be gentle.

If the needle cannot be removed because the tissue is tense, the acupuncturist may attempt removal by inserting the needle 0.1 or 0.2 chun (0.3 to 0.6 cm.) deeper and then using the push-pull method for removal.

If this method fails, insert a second acupuncture needle at a near or remote acupuncture point and perform a gentle push-pull motion for a short time. This should relax the tissues and allow removal of the original needle. If the patient shows concern at the insertion of a second needle, the acupuncturist may instead attempt to indent the skin around the point of insertion with his fingernail in the hope of relaxing the tissue and thus permitting removal of the needle.

### 10. Managing Neurogenic Shock during Acupuncture

Neurogenic shock may occur because the patient is afraid of being pierced with the needle, or the acupuncturist's technique is rough, or the patient is tired or hungry. The phenomenon often occurs during the patient's first treatment. The symptoms that usually occur after the insertion of the needle are vertigo, blurred vision, nausea, and a faint feeling. When the reaction is severe, the symptoms include pallor, cold sweats, coldness of the hands and feet, and even loss of consciousness.

*Treatment:* When the acupuncturist observes symptoms of shock the procedure should be interrupted, and it is preferable to remove the needle. In the mild case the patient should lie down and be given water to drink. He will probably recover. If the case is severe, the needle must be extracted and the patient placed in the recumbent position. The acupuncturist should press point 14.11 with his finger; the patient should regain consciousness. When he does, let him drink some warm water. If the pulse is not palpable, acupuncture needles should be inserted on the face at 14.11 and on the dorsum of each foot at 12.3. At the same time artificial respiration should be given. The acupuncture and respiration treatments should be continued until the pulse is palpable. The patient should be allowed to rest for a while and then given some warm broth. He will recover slowly.

If shock has occurred during insertion of the needle in the upper portion of the body, the resuscitation needles should be placed at points 3.7. If shock has resulted during insertion of needles in the lower portion of the body, insert resuscitation needles at 14.11 on the face or at 2.2.

# Section IV:
# Moxibustion Methods

## 1. Materials Used in Moxibustion

The material for moxibustion is produced by grinding dried moxa leaves in a mortar and sifting out the stems. The end product is a pale yellow fiber which can be made into cones or wicks ready for use.

a. How to make a cone: Put a pinch of moxa fiber on a flat wooden board and knead it into a cone with the thumb, index, and middle fingers (Fig. 9). The cone should be tightly kneaded to a size that depends on the location of the point of application and the nature of the illness to be treated. A small cone will be about the size of a baby green pea; a large one roughly the size of an olive seed. The cones are solid, not hollow.

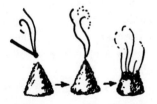

**Fig. 9**   Moxa cone and moxibustion

b. How to make a wick: The first step is to take any thin combustible paper, such as mulberry paper, and cut it into rectangles 6.0 chuns (19.0 cm.) long by 4.0 chuns (13.0 cm.) wide. Spread 6.0 chiens (22.0 grams) of moxa fiber over the paper and pat it down evenly with a spatula or small paddle. Allow a clear edge of 0.5 chun (1.6 cm.) width along the four edges of the paper and fold these edges over the layer of moxa. Next place a knitting needle or smooth wire along one of the long edges and roll a wick about the needle almost up to the opposite edge. Then clasp the wick firmly and withdraw the needle or wire. Finally, paste up the other edge so that you have a finger-size moxa wick (Fig. 10).

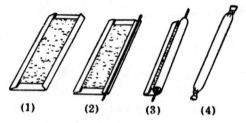

**(1)**        **(2)**        **(3)**        **(4)**

**Fig. 10**   Rolling a moxa wick

## 2. How to Perform Moxibustion

a. Direct moxibustion: Place a cone on the skin directly at the acupuncture point in question and light the tip with either a match or a stick of incense. Remove—and, if necessary, replace—the cone before it is quite burned down or when the patient complains about its heat. Dosage depends on the characteristics of the acupuncture point being used and on the nature of the illness (Fig. 9).

b. Indirect heat: To apply indirect heat, first place a slice of ginger root, onion, or some similar material on the skin at the acupuncture point, then burn the cone on top of the slice. The name applied to the method depends on the material used. The following are common bedside methods (Fig. 11):

i. Ginger moxibustion: Use a very thin (0.1 or 0.2 cm.) slice of fresh ginger which has been punctured with a needle several times. Place

16

this over the acupuncture point and burn cones, as instructed above, replacing them as the patient complains, until the skin at the acupoint is bright red. This method is especially suited for treating vomiting, diarrhea and dysentery, abdominal pain, and similar ailments, as well as illnesses that have vague symptoms and are not accompanied by fever.

*ii. Onion method:* Use the same method as before, with the ginger replaced by a thin slice of onion. This method is used for treating lockjaw in babies, for example.

*iii. Moxibustion over salt:* Used for treating abdominal pain, combined acute vomiting and diarrhea, aftereffects of blood loss in childbirth, and some cases of protruding bowel. An effective method is to fill the navel with ordinary table salt and burn cones on top of the salt.

c. How to use the wicks: Take a wick and aim it so the ignited end is toward the acupoint at a distance determined both by the patient's reaction and by the nature of the illness. The wick may be moved in and out to avoid blistering and yet make sure that sufficient heat reaches the skin surface. The duration of treatment ranges from five minutes up to half an hour. Treatment is stopped when the areas of application feel comfortably warm and show a patch of redness. Wicks are especially useful in treating such chronic ailments as indigestion, aches and pains from a cold, numbness of a treated area, etc. (Fig. 12).

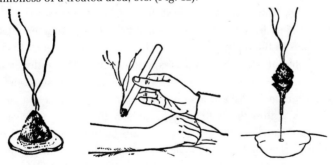

| **Fig. 11** | **Fig. 12** | **Fig. 13** |
| Indirect heating | Moxibustion with a wick | Heating through a needle |

d. Heat applied through a needle: Warm-needle moxibustion is sometimes called needle-stem moxibustion. It is usually applied during the passive phase of acupuncture. A wad of moxa fiber about the size of a date seed is placed around the top of the needle and ignited, thus transmitting heat into the acupoint through the needle. Again the dosage, in terms of the number of wads used, depends on the nature of the illness. Hot or burning ashes can be kept off the skin by placing a slightly bent piece of cardboard with a small hole over the acupoint while the needle is being applied through the hole (Fig. 13).

# Section V:
# Acupuncture Theory and the Acupuncture Points

### 1. What Is Chin Lo?

The literal meaning of *Chin* is "pathway" or "road"; *Lo* means "network." Thus, in its simplest form *Chin Lo* comprises the network of pathways within the human body connecting the internal organs to the body surface. A Chin is a kind of channel. Every major internal organ has its corresponding Chin. The pathway of this channel is permanent. Along each channel are distributed a certain number of discrete acupuncture points. The Lo is a system of pathways within the body which connect the Chins, forming a network throughout the body. The entire body is crisscrossed by this network, which encompasses all parts of the body and forms a single, unified, overall network. Thus, this network has two capabilities: (a) it transmits Ch'i fluid, and (b) it provides a route by which diseases may enter the body and reach vital organs.

The transmission of Ch'i fluid enables us to carry on ordinary life functions such as grasping with the hand, speaking, and abstract thinking. The extensiveness and complexity of the network allows this flow of Ch'i fluid to reach every part of the body. On the other hand, the network provides routes for the propagation of disease. Because the Chin Lo system connects the exterior of the body by pathways to the viscera, external factors such as cold can penetrate and produce symptoms such as coughing or abdominal pain. Similarly, diseases of internal organs will produce superficial symptoms, thus causing symptoms to reveal themselves along the skin lines.[1] For example, liver disease will cause pain in the ribs, and kidney disease will result in back pain at the waist. Thus, an analysis of superficial symptoms, conducted at the bedside, will help direct us to the appropriate internal organ and the correct combination of therapeutic acupuncture points on the skin.

It follows that the general concept of a network system through which energy flows through the body and its various parts provides the theoretical basis for the therapeutic technique commonly known as acupuncture or as acupuncture and moxibustion. The essence of the method is the administration of treatment to the specific points on the skin that are related to the internal organs by way of the system of channels. To illustrate the treatment technique, indigestion and heartburn may be treated by inserting acupuncture needles at point 3.7 on the leg, because this point is joined into the internal stomach organ system. This pathway has a skin line extending from the face downward over the chest and abdomen through the leg and terminating on the tip of the second toe. Similarly, unilateral toothache will respond to needle treatment at point 2.2, which is on the colon skin line. This line or meridian extends from the index finger, passing through the shoulder and neck, and then reaches the face. Thus, we see the importance of the theory of Chin Lo to acupuncture and moxibustion therapy. It is fundamental.

1. Skin lines are lines on the skin tracing the Chin pathways in the body.—Trans.

## 2. The Twelve Regular Chins and Their Associated Organs

Within the body there are six solid viscera—the heart, liver, spleen, lung, kidney, and pericardium; and six hollow viscera—the gallbladder, stomach, colon, small intestine, urinary bladder, and the "triple warmer." [2] Thus there are twelve internal organs. Each of these internal organs has its unique associated internal pathway (Chin).

These twelve pathways collectively are known as the regular Chins. The nomenclature for these Chins is designed to contain the names of the organ associated with the internal pathway thus named. For example, we have a heart Chin, a liver Chin, a gallbladder Chin, and a stomach Chin.

According to the Yin-Yang theory of Chinese medicine, the six solid organs are all of the Yin type: lung and spleen are most Yin; heart and kidney are least Yin; liver and pericardium are normal Yin. The six hollow viscera are of the Yang type: the small intestine and the urinary bladder are most Yang; the gallbladder and triple warmer are least Yang; the stomach and colon are normal Yang. The six skin lines associated with the six Yin internal pathways corresponding to the solid organs all lie on the inner side (the Yin side) of the extremities and, in the same fashion, the six skin lines associated with the Yang pathways of the hollow organs all lie on the outer (Yang) surfaces of the arms and legs. Furthermore, since each internal pathway, and thus its associated skin line, passes along an extremity, these pathways are identified as being either arm pathways (the three arm/Yin and the three arm/Yang pathways) or leg pathways (the three leg/Yin and the three leg/Yang pathways). These twelve pathways, the regular Chins, are also sometimes called the twelve Chin vessels to distinguish them from the vessels to be introduced in the next section.

The skin lines corresponding to the twelve regular Chins fall into four categories:

2. The "triple warmer" is a hypothetical organ which has no known anatomical entity.—Trans.

a. The three Yin skin lines of the arm:

   Arm/most Yin/lung, Arm/normal Yin/pericardium, Arm/least
   Yin/heart

These three skin lines all originate on the chest and travel along the
Yin surface of the arm to the fingers.

b. The three Yang skin lines of the arm:

   Arm/normal Yang/colon, Arm/least Yang/triple warmer, Arm/
   most Yang/small intestine

These three skin lines all begin on the fingers and travel along the
Yang surface of the arm, terminating on the head.

c. The three Yang skin lines of the leg:

   Leg/normal Yang/stomach, Leg/least Yang/gallbladder, Leg/
   most Yang/urinary bladder

These three lines all originate on the head, pass down the back, and
twirl downward to reach the legs on the front, lateral, and posterior
surfaces, respectively.

d. The three Yin skin lines of the leg:

   Leg/most Yin/spleen, Leg/normal Yin/liver, Leg/least Yin/
   kidney

These lines originate on the toes, traverse the inner surfaces of the
legs, and terminate on either the abdomen or the chest.

In addition to the methods of classifying the twelve regular Chins
just considered, it is equally important to take into account the fact
that they occur in pairs. Among the twelve Chins, every Yin Chin is
paired with a Yang Chin, its opposite. That is to say, the lines tend to
fall naturally into pairs which follow roughly comparable paths
along opposing Yin and Yang body surfaces, and in fact may be
considered to have actual internal connections near or on the fingers
or toes, as the case may be. This matching into pairs is known in
Chinese medicine as *Piao-Li* matching (or, at times, Yin-Yang
matching). The two organs that correspond to the two elements of a
pair influence one another (as shown in the table below). Thus, at
the bedside, a point on a given skin line may be used not only to treat
ailments associated with that skin line, but also to treat illnesses
associated with its matching skin line. For example, the arm/normal

21

Yang/colon line is paired with the line of the arm/most Yin/lung. Therefore point 1.1 on the lung line may be used not only to treat a cough; it may also be involved in the treatment of dysentery. Similarly, since leg/most Yin/spleen is paired with leg/normal Yang/stomach, point 3.7 on the stomach line can be used not only in connection with indigestion and heart burn—it is also useful in treating diarrhea. These examples serve to illustrate the close relationship between each Yin pathway and its corresponding Yang pathway.

Table 1. Piao-Li (Yin-Yang) Matching Pairs

Arm/most Yin/lung—Arm/normal Yang/colon
Arm/least Yin/heart—Arm/most Yang/small intestine
Arm/normal Yin/pericardium—Arm/least Yang/triple warmer
Leg/most Yin/spleen—Leg/normal Yang/stomach
Leg/least Yin/kidney—Leg/most Yang/urinary bladder
Leg/normal Yin/liver—Leg/least Yang/gallbladder

### 3. The Other Eight Chins

The eight Chin vessels differ from the twelve regular Chins in that no one of them is associated with a specific organ. On the contrary, they crisscross and pass through various regular Chins and thus have only indirect organ relationships. In this sense these eight Chins differ from the regular Chins; thus they are sometimes referred to as irregular Chins.[3]

Altogether there are eight irregular Chins: Tu vessel (governing vessel), Jen vessel (vessel of conception), Chung vessel, Tai vessel, Yin Chiao, Yang Chiao, Yin Wei, and Yang Wei. The first two of these vessels—the governing vessel and the vessel of conception—have their skin lines on the midline of the body, anterior and posterior respectively. Each of the two has a specific set of acupuncture points. The other six internal pathways have no associated body

3. They are also sometimes called extra meridians.—Trans.

points, and thus no skin lines. Their relationship with the twelve regular Chins is internal. Thus, the first two of the vessels are those of greatest significance to acupuncture. They are frequently grouped with the twelve regular Chins to collectively constitute the fourteen Chin pathways.

## 4. The Fourteen Pathways—Associated Symptoms and Initial and Terminal Points

We have already explained that each of the fourteen pathways has associated skin lines. Each also has a definite initial point and a definite terminal. We have also mentioned that diseases of internal organs will produce superficial symptoms. In the following discussion we will explain in specific terms how the skin lines are associated with the internal pathways and related disorders.

### ONE: ARM/MOST YIN/LUNG

On each skin line there are eleven points and, since the skin line is bilateral, there are twenty-two body points in all. The line originates on the chest at the point Chungfu, on the third rib at the upper part of the breast. The line passes along the inner surface of the arm and terminates on the radial edge of the thumb tip at 1.4. The internal pathway is connected to arm/normal Yang/colon.

*Therapeutic usage:* Labored breathing or shortness of breath, coughing, pressure and swelling in the chest area, and pain on the anterior of the shoulders.

### TWO: ARM/NORMAL YANG/COLON

There are twenty points on each side, forty in all. The skin line originates on the radial side of the index finger at 2.1, on the tip, and moves along the lateral surface of the arm along the shoulder and neck to a termination at 2.5 at the side of the nose. It is connected internally to the leg/normal Yang/stomach Chin.

*Therapeutic usage:* Abdominal pain, dryness in the mouth, toothache, nosebleed, clear nasal discharge, sore throat, pain on the lateral side of the shoulder, and pain at the index finger.

### Three: Leg/Normal Yang/Stomach

Each skin line contains forty-five points, ninety in all. Beginning at Chengchi below the eye, the line passes across the cheek and follows the contours of the lips to the chinbone, thence backward and slightly downward, and then divides into two branches. One of these branches moves upward past the front of the ear and then through the hairline to terminate at 3.4 on the horn of the forehead (the frontal eminence). The other branch moves downward along the neck and over the chest, abdomen, and frontal ridge of the thigh to a terminus at 3.11 on the tip of the second toe at the corner of the nail nearest the little toe. It is internally connected to leg/most Yin/spleen.

*Therapeutic usage:* Pressure and swelling in the abdomen, heartburn and indigestion, vomiting, nosebleed, facial distortion, and high fever.

### Four: Leg/Most Yin/Spleen

On each side there are twenty-one points, forty-two in all. The skin line originates at point 4.1 on the tip of the big toe along the edge away from the other toes. The line moves upward along the inner side of the leg near the anterior and farther upward to the chest to terminate at the point Tapao on the ribs. Internal connection is to arm/least Yin/heart.

*Therapeutic usage:* Pressure and swelling in the abdomen, indigestion and heartburn, vomiting, diarrhea, and coldness along the inner thigh.

### Five: Arm/Least Yin/Heart

Each skin line contains nine points, eighteen in all. The line begins near the armpit at Chichuan and moves along the ulnar side of the inner surface of the arm to terminate near the tip of the little finger on the radial edge. The internal connection is to arm/most Yang/small intestine.

*Therapeutic usage:* Dry throat, thirst, pain near the heart, and aching along the ribs or inner arm.

## Six: Arm/Most Yang/Small Intestine

On each side there are nineteen points, thirty-eight in all. The origin is 6.1 at the ulnar edge of the little finger. The line traverses the arm on the lateral surface along the posterior and up the neck to terminate at 6.3 in front of the ear near the tragus. The interior connection is to leg/most Yang/urinary bladder.

*Therapeutic usage:* Deafness, yellow eyes, swollen neck, and pain in the neck and along the anterior of the upper arm.

## Seven: Leg/Most Yang/Urinary Bladder

There are sixty-seven points on each side, altogether one hundred and thirty-four. The skin line commences at point 7.1 near the inner corner of the eye, moves upward across the top of the head, down the neck and alongside the spine past the back of the waist and over the hip, proceeds down the back of the leg, curves around the outer ankle and along the outer edge of the foot to a termination at point 7.12 on the outer tip of the little toe. It is internally connected to leg/least Yin/kidney.

*Therapeutic usage:* Headache, pain along the spine, pain at the back of the waist, pain in the legs and feet, cramps in the calf, and malaria.

## Eight: Leg/Least Yin/Kidney

Twenty-seven points lie on each side, to make a total of fifty-four points. The line begins at point 8.1, which is at the cavity in the center of the sole of the foot. Moving upward, the line traverses the inner side of the leg, passes over the abdomen, and terminates at Shufu on the chest. The internal connection is with arm/normal Yin/pericardium.

*Therapeutic usage:* Coughing, coughing up or vomiting blood, labored breathing or shortness of breath, dry tongue, and pain at the back of the waist.

## Nine: Arm/Normal Yin/Pericardium

There are nine points per side, eighteen in all. The skin line begins about one body chun to the outside of the nipple at the point Tien-chih, passes through the central portion of the lateral surface of the arm, and terminates at point 9.4 on the tip of the middle finger. It connects internally with arm/least Yang/triple warmer.

*Therapeutic usage:* Pressure and swelling in the chest region, irregular pulse, mental depression, vomiting, stupor, and throbbing pain of the upper arm.

### TEN: ARM/LEAST YANG/TRIPLE WARMER

There are twenty-three points on each side, forty-six in all. Origin is at the ulnar edge of the tip of the ring finger at point 10.1. The line moves up the arm on the center of the lateral surface, up the neck, past the back of the ear, and terminates at point 10.7 on the outer tip of the eyebrow. Internal connection is to leg/least Yang/gallbladder.

*Therapeutic usage:* Headache, pain of the eye, deafness, sore throat, and pain on the outer side of the upper arm and shoulder.

### ELEVEN: LEG/LEAST YANG/GALLBLADDER

Forty-four points lie on each side, so there are eighty-eight in all. The line originates at Tungtzuliao near the outer corner of the eye, passes along the temple and behind the ear and downward across the neck and shoulder, the side of the chest, the abdomen, the hip, and the outside of the leg, and terminates at point 11.6 on the tip of the fourth toe. It connects with leg/normal Yin/liver.

*Therapeutic usage:* Headache, pain at the outer corner of the eye socket, pain in the chest area, and pain on the outer side of the knee.

### TWELVE: LEG/NORMAL YIN/LIVER

Each side contains fourteen points, for a total of twenty-eight. The skin line begins at point 12.1 on the tip of the big toe along the edge nearest the second toe, moves upward along the inner surface of the leg and over the abdomen, to terminate at Chimen on the chest below the breast. The vessel connects internally to arm/most Yin/lung.

*Therapeutic usage:* Lower abdominal pain during pregnancy, pain at the back of the waist, liquid stools, inability to urinate, and bed-wetting.

### Thirteen: The Vessel of Conception

This line contains twenty-four points. The line begins at Huiyin, midway between the anus and the genitals, proceeds upward through the pubic hair and along the midline of the abdomen and straight up to the throat area, and terminates at point 13.7 in the central cavity between the chin and the lower lip. It is connected internally to the governing vessel.

*Therapeutic usage:* Pain in the lower abdomen, inability to urinate, and bed-wetting.

### Fourteen: The Governing Vessel

There are twenty-eight points on the skin line. It begins at point 14.1 below the coccyx and moves upward right along the middle of the spine and the back of the neck and over the top of the head, passes along the ridge of the nose to arrive at the lip and terminate at Yinchiao on the inner surface of the upper lip. There it connects internally with both the vessel of conception and with leg/normal Yang/stomach.

*Therapeutic usage:* Stiffness and inability to bend the back.

# Section VI:
# The Acupuncture Points

## 1. What Is an Acupuncture Point?

An acupuncture point is simply a point at which one of the internal channels (Chin) comes into proximity with the skin surface and thus is a point where external influences can be transmitted to internal organs. These are then the points at which acupuncture and moxibustion are administered. Though there are many of these points on the body surface, their classification falls into three simple categories: the pathway points, the isolated points, and the "ouch" points. Whenever a point lies on any one of the fourteen pathways—which is to say it has a fixed location on one of the fourteen skin lines—it is called the pathway point and is given a specific name. Isolated points are points that fail to lie on any of the skin lines but which, through clinical experience, have been shown to have therapeutic value. The "ouch" points also fail to lie on any of the skin lines, but they have also been shown through clinical experience to have therapeutic value. They have no specific location. During a period of illness certain areas of the body will tend to become tender, especially when subjected to finger pressure. The number and location of these "ouch" points will vary according to the nature of the illness. These points are useful in treating superficial pain (such as in a pulled muscle) and also serve as supplementary points to increase the effectiveness of therapy applied at pathway points.

## 2. How to Locate a Point

Acupuncture points are widely distributed over the body surface. The effectiveness of treatment is directly dependent on precision and skill in locating these points. There are three commonly used methods for determining these locations.

a. Location through recognition of body features. This method is not only simple and convenient but it is also highly accurate. It is therefore the preferred method for bedside use. For example, point 15.1 can be found directly between the eyebrows; 1.2 can be found by having the patient slide his hands together and observing where his index finger reaches the small cavity between the bones of the forearm. The point 13.6 lies on the midline of the body halfway between the two breasts; point 14.3 lies on the spine directly behind the navel. Using a method which we will describe later, the vertebrae form landmarks that locate certain points such as 14.6 on the first vertebra and 14.5 on the second vertebra (employing the method of enumeration which we will describe later on in conjunction with methods for locating 7.3).

b. Location using the middle finger as a unit of measurement. The body chun is a useful unit of measurement since it takes into account the specifics of the body habitus. The middle finger chun is an appropriate lateral unit to use when locating points on the arms and legs and on the upper back. This unit of length is determined by placing the tip of the patient's middle finger against his thumb tip to form a ring, and then determining the distance between the wrinkles at the first and second joints of the middle finger in the same manner shown in Figure 14.

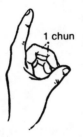

**Fig. 14**   Measuring 1 body chun on the middle finger

c. Methods based on skeletal measurements. In this method a fixed number of units is assigned to the distance between two given body locations. This system of attributing a certain number of units of distance between two given body features is applicable to any patient, male or female, old or young, tall or short, obese or slim. The following are the most common systems in current use (Fig. 15):

i. *Head body chun (lateral):* Assign a measure of 9 units to the distance between the corners of the jaws (angles of the mandible). One of these units is then 1 body chun.

ii. *Head body chun (longitudinal):* Assign a measure of 12 units to the distance along the midline of the head from the hairline over the forehead to the hairline at the back of the neck. If the back hairline is not easily distinguishable, measure instead to 14.6 and assign 3 additional units to the total distance, thus assigning 15 units. If the front hairline cannot be determined, measure instead from a point directly between the eyebrows to the hairline on the neck and assign

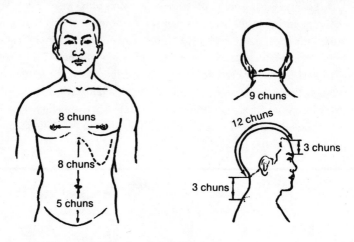

**Fig. 15**  Skeletal body chuns

3 additional units, 15 in all. If neither hairline is visible, assign 18 units to the distance from 14.6 to the point between the brows.

*iii. Chest and abdomen body chun (lateral):* Assign 8 units to the distance between the two nipples.

*iv. Chest body chun (longitudinal):* The distance separating two alternate ribs is assigned the value of 1.6 body chuns.

*v. Upper abdominal body chun (longitudinal):* The distance between the lower tip of the sternum and the navel is assigned a value of 8 units.

*vi. Lower abdominal body chun (longitudinal):* From the navel to the pubis (the horizontal prominence in the pelvic area) is assigned 5 units.

*vii. Back body chun (longitudinal):* A measure of 30 units is assigned to the distance from the first vertebra (thoracic vertebra I) to the twenty-first vertebra (coccyx). This method is infrequent in practice, since the vertebrae themselves serve as marking points.

*viii. Back body chun (lateral):* The middle finger body chun serves

as a lateral unit for the back as well as both a lateral and a longitudinal unit for use on the arms and legs.

## 3. How to Form Curative Combinations

The practice of acupuncture and moxibustion closely resembles
the practice of medicine in that the therapist must base his decisions
on the physical makeup of the patient and the nature of the illness
—severe or mild, acute or chronic. Curative combinations of points
must be selected at the bedside, and effectiveness of the treatment
depends on this choice. There are certain fixed rules that will assist
in making a proper selection, a few of which are given here:

a. Points along the primary pathway: When locating points along
the primary skin line associated with a given illness, it is customary
to choose points below the elbow (if an arm line) or knee (if a leg
line). If, for example, the illness involves the nose, the associated
skin line will be the arm/normal Yang/colon line, applying the
needle at 2.2; for heart trouble the two normal Yin lines are primary,
and 9.3 is a natural choice; stomach trouble is related to the leg/
normal Yang line, and 3.7 is a typical choice. In short, this technique
is based on selecting remote points along the proper skin line.

b. Points near the site of the ailment: This method involves
choosing points close to the site of the ailment. Here the choice is
based on proximity rather than on skin line. For example, headache
may be treated at points 14.8, 11.2, 14.9, and 15.2, all of which are on
the head. Shoulder pain may direct the choice of 2.4 and 2.3. For
pain at the back of the waist, 7.8 or 11.3 may be indicated. And 7.1
and 7.2 may be the choice in treating an eye disorder. Thus the
treatment is based on choices of nearby points.

c. Points that match: After a point has been selected for
acupuncture, it may be deemed advisable to choose one or two
related points in order to improve the effectiveness of the therapy.
Since this matching of points is a very common bedside procedure,
several means of doing this will be described.

i. *Matching remote points with nearby points:* This is a combination of methods (a) and (b) as just described. As an example, the

remote point 3.7 is appropriate for treating stomach disorders, while 13.5 is an indicated nearby point. For nose problems the remote point 2.2 may be paired with the nearby 2.5. For painful menstruation, pair the remote point 12.3 with the nearby point 13.2. For eye disorders the remote point is 6.2 and the proximal point is 7.1.

*ii. Choosing bilateral pairs:* The method is to select a proper point and then also choose its bilateral counterpart. In stomach problems, for instance, both of the points 3.7 or both of 9.3 may be selected. For headache either the pair 15.2 or the pair 1.2 may be used. For female disorders either the pair 4.2 or the pair 4.4 may be treated.

*iii. Arm and leg pairing:* It is possible to pair a point on the arm with one on the leg, or vice versa. For instance, 9.3 may be paired with 3.7 to treat stomach or intestinal problems; 5.2 may be matched with 4.2 in treating insomnia; pain along the ribs suggests pairing 10.5 with 11.4; 2.2 and 3.10 may be combined in treating toothache; and 10.5 may be paired with 8.3 to form a curative combination for constipation.

*iv. Front and back pairing:* Front and back matching, or echoing, involves pairing a point on the front part of the body with one on the back part. As an example, nasal congestion may be treated by matching 2.5 with 11.2.

*v. Piao-Li or Yin-Yang matching:* This method consists of matching each Yin pathway with its corresponding Yang pathway. For instance, to treat colds or influenza, 2.2 on the colon line may be matched with 1.2 on the lung line; for indigestion, match 3.7 on the stomach line with 4.2 on the spleen line.

*vi. Chain matching:* Select an appropriate arm or leg skin line and, on one side of the body only, choose two or three points that are well separated and form a chain along the limb. For example, 2.4, 2.3, and 2.2 may be chosen to treat pain in the arm; 11.3, 11.4, and 11.5 may be used to treat paralysis on one side of the body.

## 4. Catalogue of Commonly Used Acupuncture Points

Altogether there are 361 points along the fourteen skin lines, and almost 600 other points are presently known which do not lie on the traditional skin lines. We are now going to describe ninety-seven of these points, eighty-four of which are on the traditional skin lines, and thirteen of which are not.

### One: Arm/Most Yin/Lung

Eleven points are known to lie along this line, four of which are within the scope of this book.

1.1 Chihtse

*Site:* In the elbow cavity at the center of the wrinkle.

*How to locate:* Seat the patient upright, arm horizontal and slightly bent at the elbow, palm up. Along the wrinkle of the elbow a large muscle can be felt (pronator teres). To the outside of this muscle (thumb side), slight finger pressure will reveal a cavity; this is the point (Fig. 16).

*Associated treatment:* Penetrate perpendicularly to a depth of 0.3 to 0.5 chun (1.0 to 1.6 cm.). Normally an aching, numb sensation will travel to the fingers along the outside of the forearm. Moxibustion dosage is five cones or five minutes with a wick.

*Associated illnesses:* Colds and flu, coughing, excessive mucus from the chest, whooping cough, and aching in the arm or elbow.

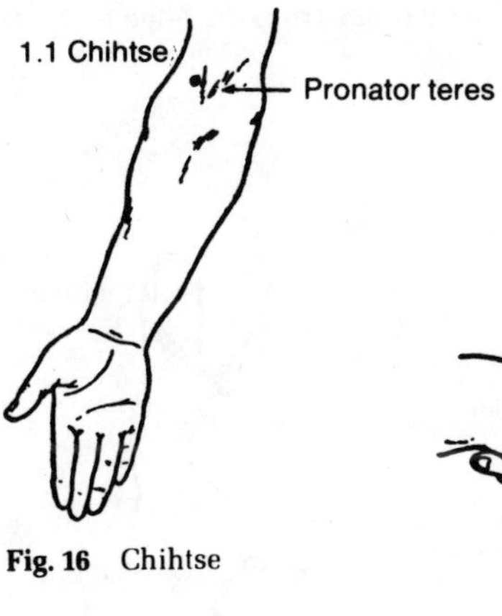

1.1 Chihtse — Pronator teres

1.2 Liehchueh

**Fig. 16** Chihtse 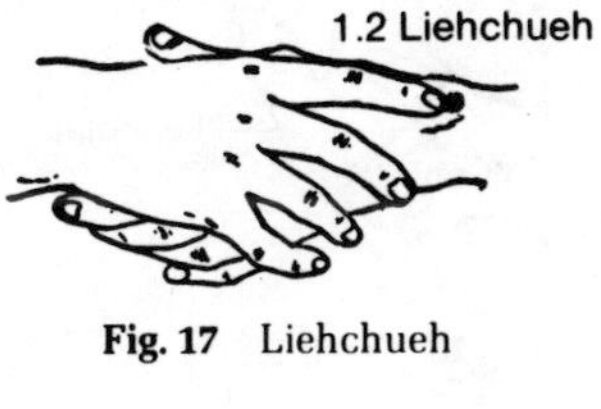    **Fig. 17** Liehchueh

### 1.2 Liehchueh

*Site:* On the forearm on the thumb side (radial aspect), 1.5 body chuns up the arm from the top of the high bone (styloid process of the radius) of the wrist.

*How to locate:* Seat the patient upright and, with the thumb and index finger of each hand spread slightly apart and straight, have the patient slide his hands together until the webs touch and one index finger lies along the radial aspect of the opposing arm. The tip of the index finger will just reach to a small cavity along the bone; this is the point (Fig. 17).

*Associated treatment:* Penetrate slightly off the perpendicular so that the needle point is angled toward the cavity of the elbow. The depth is between 0.2 and 0.3 chun (0.6 to 1.0 cm.). Normally an aching, numb sensation will travel to the fingers along the outside of the forearm. Moxibustion dosage is seven cones or five minutes with a wick.

*Associated illnesses:* Colds and flu, headache, coughing, aching in the wrist, toothache, and facial distortion.

### 1.3 Yuchi

*Site:* On the palm between the thumb and the wrist.

*How to locate:* Seat the patient upright, palm up. Draw an imaginary line from the center of the palm to a point of the radial aspect midway along the bone connecting the thumb and the wrist. Locate a point one-fourth of the distance from the edge to the center; this is the point (Fig. 18).

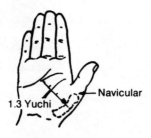

**Fig. 18** Yuchi

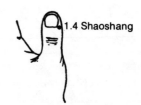

**Fig. 19** Shaoshang

*Associated treatment:* Insertion should be perpendicular to a depth of 0.3 to 0.5 chun (1.0 to 1.6 cm.). Moxibustion dosage is three cones or five minutes with a wick.

*Associated illnesses:* Fever, coughing, pain in the chest or ribs, and sore throat.

1.4 Shaoshang

*Site:* About 0.1 body chun from the corner of the base of the thumbnail in the radial direction.

*How to locate:* Seat the patient upright, with the fist slightly clenched and the thumb straight atop the index finger. The point lies on the radial edge of the thumb at a distance of about 0.1 body chun from the corner of the base of the nail (Fig. 19).

*Associated treatment:* Penetrate at an angle, needle tip aimed toward the knuckle to a depth of 0.1 chun (0.3 cm.). Frequently this point is a site for letting one or two drops of blood with a trocar needle.

*Associated illnesses:* Nosebleeds, vomiting, sore throat, pinkeye, whooping cough, epilepsy, and stroke.


Two: ARM/NORMAL YANG/COLON

Of the twenty points along this line, five are discussed here.

2.1 Shangyang

*Site:* On the radial aspect (the side closest to the thumb) of the index finger about 0.1 body chun from the corner of the base of the nail.

*How to locate:* Seat the patient upright and have him point with his index finger with thumb pointed up, other three fingers folded. The point is located about 0.1 body chun up from the corner of the base of the nail (Fig. 20).

*Associated treatment:* Same as 1.4. Moxibustion dosage is three cones or five minutes with a wick.

*Associated illnesses:* Whooping cough, pinkeye, and stroke.

2.2 Hoku

*Site:* On the back of the hand between the first and second bones.

*How to locate:* Seat the patient upright and select the hand on

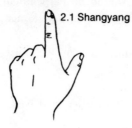

2.1 Shangyang

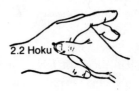

2.2 Hoku

**Fig. 20**  Shangyang            **Fig. 21**  Hoku

which the point is to be located. Have the patient extend the thumb and index finger of this hand, angled apart; place the thumb of his other hand, palm down, over the back of the first hand so that the wrinkle across the knuckle of the thumb of the second hand coincides exactly with the edge of the web between the thumb and the index finger of the first hand. The point lies beneath the tip of this second thumb, slightly toward the index finger (Fig. 21).

*Associated treatment:* Use perpendicular penetration (needle tip canted slightly in the direction of the arm) to a depth of 0.5 to 0.8 chun (1.6 to 2.6 cm.); a sensation of numbness will sometimes travel both up the arm and down toward the fingers. Needles may not be applied at this point if the patient is pregnant. Moxibustion dosage is three cones or five to seven minutes with a wick.

*Associated illnesses:* Colds and flu, fever, coughing, vomiting, headache, toothache, sore throat, sinus trouble (ill-smelling nasal discharge), heatstroke, cholera, stroke, whooping cough, pinkeye, deafness, mumps, painful menstruation, failure to menstruate, difficult childbirth, aching wrist, boils, and facial distortion.

2.3 Chuchih

*Site:* On the ulnar aspect near the wrinkle of the elbow.

*How to locate:* Seat the patient upright, arm bent at a right angle. The point lies midway between the terminus of the wrinkle of the elbow and the peak of the high bone (head of the radius) (Fig. 22).

*Associated treatment:* Use perpendicular penetration to a depth of 0.8 to 1.5 chuns (2.6 to 4.8 cm.). The patient will sometime sense aching and numbness in the hands and arms. Moxibustion dosage is three to seven cones or five to ten minutes with a wick.

*Associated illnesses:* Colds and flu, fever, vomiting, heatstroke, cramps or spasms in the limbs, epilepsy, pain in the gums, mumps, aches in the shoulders and elbows, and skin rash.

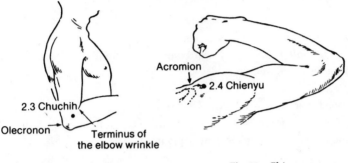

**Fig. 22**  Chuchih          **Fig. 23**  Chienyu

2.4 Chienyu

*Site:* On the tip of the shoulder at the joint.

*How to locate:* Raise the patient's arm to a horizontal position and note the cavity that lies on the upper arm, 1.0 body chun from the tip of the shoulder (acromion); this is the point (Fig. 23).

*Associated treatment:* Apply perpendicular penetration to a depth of 0.6 to 1.0 chun (1.9 to 3.2 cm.). For moxibustion apply ten cones or use wicks for ten to fifteen minutes.

*Associated illness:* Aching in the shoulder area.

2.5 Yinghsian

*Site:* On the cheek, outside of the nose, near the nostril.

*How to locate:* Seat the patient upright. Starting at the outside edge of the nose at the nostril, go out by 0.5 body chun; this is the point (Fig. 24).

*Associated treatment:* Enter from a perpendicular direction to a depth of 0.3 chun (1.0 cm.). Moxibustion is forbidden at this point.

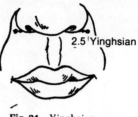

**Fig. 24** Yinghsian

*Associated illnesses:* Nasal congestion, windburned eyes, sinus trouble, colds, and flu.

THREE: LEG/NORMAL YANG/STOMACH

There are forty-five body points along this skin line. We describe the eleven that are most commonly used.

3.1 Titsang

*Site:* Near the corner of the mouth.

*How to locate:* Seat the patient, either upright or on a chair with a headrest. Visualize two lines, the first running horizontally out from the corner of the mouth and the second being the facial fold bending downward from the nose above and alongside the mouth. At the intersection of these two lines, about 0.4 body chun from the corner of the mouth, lies the point (Fig. 25).

*Associated treatment:* Insert with the needle point slanted toward the earlobe to a depth of 0.3 to 0.5 chun (1.0 to 1.6 cm.). Moxibustion dosage is five cones or five minutes with a wick.

*Associated illness:* Facial distortion.

3.2 Chiache

*Site:* Forward of the angle of the jawbone.

*How to locate:* Seat the patient upright or with head leaning back. Move forward and up from the lower back corner of the jawbone for a distance of about 0.8 body chun. Have the patient close his mouth and lips tightly and bite down, thus causing his chewing muscle (masseter) to protrude outward. The highest point along this muscle is particularly sensitive to finger pressure to the extent of its being painful; this is the point (Fig. 25).

*Associated treatment:* Either penetrate from the perpendicular to a depth of 0.4 chun (1.4 cm.) or at a slant in the direction of 3.1. Moxibustion dosage is three to five cones or five to seven minutes with a wick.

*Associated illnesses:* Facial distortion, toothache, epilepsy, and mumps.

3.3 Hsiakuan

*Site:* In front of the tragus (the little ear).

*How to locate:* Seat the patient upright and have him close his mouth. Press the finger at the base of the tragus and move forward horizontally for a distance of 0.7 to 0.8 body chun. A cavity can be felt here while the mouth is closed, but the area puffs up as the mouth is opened; this is the point (Fig. 25).

*Associated treatment:* Penetrate from the perpendicular to a depth of 0.3 chun (1.0 cm.). Do *not* apply moxibustion at this point.

*Associated illnesses:* Facial distortion and toothache.

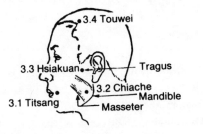

**Fig. 25**   Titsang, Chiache, Hsiakuan, and Touwei        **Fig. 26**   Touwei

3.4 Touwei

*Site:* Above the hairline on the extension of the line joining the prominence of the forehead to the corner.

*How to locate:* Seat the patient upright. Starting at the central point between the eyebrows, go up vertically a distance of 0.5 body chun and then measure outward a distance of 4.5 body chuns. Starting from here, move up to the corner of the hairline and a distance of 0.5 body chun beyond; this is the point (Figs. 25 and 26).

*Associated treatment:* Needle penetration should be parallel to the skin contour in the direction of the top of the head; depth is 0.3 chun (1.0 cm.). Do *not* apply moxibustion to this point.

*Associated illnesses:* Headache, headache along the temples, and aching behind the ridge of the eyebrow.

3.5 Tienshu

*Site:* On either side of the navel.

*How to locate:* Have the patient lie on his back. Measure from the navel outward to the left, or right, a distance of 2.0 body chuns. Here, horizontal to the navel, are the points (Fig. 27).

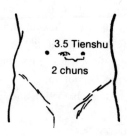

**Fig. 27**   Tienshu

*Associated treatment:* Penetrate from the perpendicular to a depth of 0.5 to 1.0 chun (1.6 to 3.2 cm.). Moxibustion dosage is seven to fifteen cones or five to fifteen minutes with wicks.

*Associated illnesses:* Abdominal pain, dysentery, cholera, irregular menstruation, bloody stools, and diarrhea.

3.6 Tupi

*Site:* At the juncture of the kneecap and the upper end of the shinbone (tibia).

*How to locate:* Seat the patient upright with his legs bent at the knee, feet dangling. Just below the kneecap and outward, there is a cavity (called the outer eye of the knee). The point is located at the center of this cavity (Fig. 29).

*Associated treatment:* The needle tip should be slanted slightly inward; depth is 0.3 to 0.4 chun (1.0 to 1.3 cm.). Moxibustion dosage is three cones or five to ten minutes with a wick.

*Associated illness:* Aching of the knee joint.

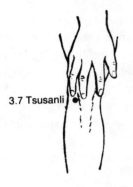

Fig. 28  Tsusanli

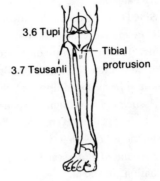

Fig. 29  Tupi and Tsusanli

3.7 Tsusanli

*Site:* Below the knee and outward.

*How to locate:* Either seat the patient upright with his feet dangling or have him lie on his back with his legs straight. Have the patient place his hand over his knee with the center of his palm over the highest point of the kneecap. Measure outward 1.0 body chun from the tip of his middle finger (Fig. 28). As an alternative method, run a finger downward from the center of the knee along the forward edge of the leg until the protruding high bone (tibial protrusion) is felt. Below this protusion, measure outward 1.0 body chun; this is the point (Fig. 29).

*Associated treatment:* Penetration should be perpendicular to a depth of 0.5 to 1.0 chun (1.6 to 3.2 cm.). This frequently will cause aching and numbness in the area, and these will ultimately spread to the instep. Sometimes the pain will move along a line to the third and fourth toes; sometimes it will travel up toward the abdomen. Moxibustion dosage is from seven cones to ten or more. Wicks should be used for thirty minutes.

*Associated illnesses:* Abdominal pain, vomiting, cholera, dysentery, inability to urinate, constipation, aches and pains in the legs, toothache, heatstroke, dizziness and nausea, appendicitis, irregular menstruation, painful menstruation, and failure to menstruate.

### 3.8 Fenglung

*Site:* Halfway down the lower leg on the outer surface.

*How to locate:* Seat the patient upright, knees bent and feet dangling. Find the midpoint of the line joining the tip of the ankle to 11.4 (below the knee joint on the outer surface). Move 1.0 body chun forward from this midpoint; this is the point (Fig. 30).

*Associated treatment:* Perpendicular penetration to a depth of 0.3 to 0.8 chun (1.0 to 2.6 cm.). Moxibustion dosage is three cones or five to ten minutes with a wick.

*Associated illnesses:* Excessive discharge from the chest, constipation, and stroke.

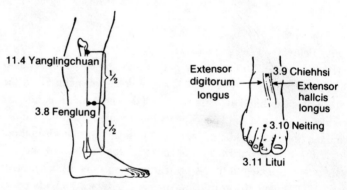

**Fig. 30** Fenglung     **Fig. 31** Chiehhsi. Neiting. and Litui

### 3.9 Chiehhsi

*Site:* At the joint between the leg and instep, front and center.

*How to locate:* Seat the patient upright with his feet flat on the floor. Above the instep in the wrinkled area (the horizontal crease near the ankle) there are two tendons (extensor digitorum longus and extensor hallucis longus). The point lies in the center of the cavity between these tendons (Fig. 31).

*Associated treatment:* Insert from the perpendicular in the direction of the heel to a depth of 0.5 to 0.8 chun (1.6 to 2.6 cm.). Moxibustion dosage is five cones or five to ten minutes with a wick.

*Associated illnesses:* Sprained ankle and vomiting.

3.10 Neiting

*Site:* Above the crevice between the second and third toes.

*How to locate:* Seat the patient upright with his feet flat. The point is on the upper surface of the foot, slightly above the crevice between the second and third toes (Fig. 31).

*Associated treatment:* Perpendicular penetration to a depth of 0.3 to 0.5 chun (1.0 to 1.6 cm.). Moxibustion dosage is three cones or five minutes with a wick.

*Associated illnesses:* Toothache in the upper teeth, sore throat, constipation, painful menstruation, and insomnia.

3.11 Litui

*Site:* On the second toe at the corner of the nail toward the little toe.

*How to locate:* Seat the patient upright, feet flat on the floor. On the second toe, locate the corner at the root of the nail and toward the little toe. Approximately 0.1 body chun away from the corner in the direction of the little toe lies the point.

*Associated treatment:* Needle depth is 0.1 chun (0.3 cm.). Moxibustion dosage is three cones or five minutes with a wick.

*Associated illnesses:* Appendicitis and unconsciousness.

FOUR: LEG/MOST YIN/SPLEEN

There are twenty known points on this skin line; four of them are described here.

4.1 Yinpai

*Site:* Near the base of the big toenail on the side away from the other toes.

*How to locate:* Seat the patient upright, feet flat on the floor. The point is 0.1 body chun away from the corner of the big toenail, away from the toes and at the base of the nail (Fig. 32).

*Associated treatment:* Needle depth is 0.1 chun (0.3 cm.). Moxibustion dosage is three cones or five minutes with a wick.

*Associated illnesses:* Irregular menstruation, heavy menstruation, insomnia, and unconsciousness.

4.2 Sanyinchiao

*Site:* On the inner surface of the leg above the ankle (inner ankle) just behind the shinbone (tibia).

*How to locate:* Seat the patient upright with his knees bent and feet dangling; or lay the patient on his back with his legs straight. Holding the index, middle, and ring fingers together, press down in the depression above the ankle, behind the tibia on the inner surface to locate a cavity; this cavity is the point (Fig. 32).

*Associated treatment:* Perpendicular insertion to a depth of 0.3 to 0.5 chun (1.0 to 1.6 cm.). Needles may not be used at this point when the patient is pregnant. Moxibustion dosage is three cones or five to ten minutes with a wick.

*Associated illnesses:* Irregular menstruation, extended menstruation, abdominal pain, painful menstruation, heavy menstruation, difficult childbirth, consequences of loss of blood in childbirth, stroke, insomnia, and bed-wetting.

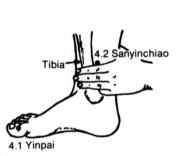

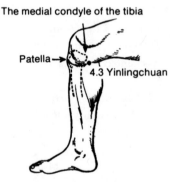

**Fig. 32**   Yinpai and Sanyinchiao          **Fig. 33**   Yinlingchuan

4.3 Yinlingchuan

*Site:* On the inner side of the lower leg behind the upper extremity of the tibia and slightly above 11.4.

*How to locate:* Seat the patient upright, legs bent and feet dangling, or supine with legs straight. Measure downward from the top of the kneecap along the ridge of the tibia until the initial portion of the prominence is felt, and then move along the inner surface in the posterior direction for a distance of 4.0 body chuns. This point, which lies between the end of the knee wrinkle and the posterior surface of the upper extremity of the tibia, is the point (Fig. 33).

*Associated treatment:* Perpendicular penetration to a depth of 0.8 chun (2.6 cm.). Moxibustion dosage is three cones or a wick for five minutes.

*Associated illnesses:* Swelling of the abdomen and pains and swelling in the knees and legs.

4.4 Hsuehhai

*Site:* On the inner surface of the thigh about 2 body chuns above the knee.

*How to locate:* Seat the patient upright, knees bent, feet dangling. Face the patient and place hand on the patient's knee with the center of the palm over the tip of the kneecap. Where the tip of the thumb touches the inner surface, this is the point (Fig. 34).

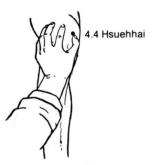

4.4 Hsuehhai

**Fig. 34**  Hsuehhai

*Associated treatment:* Perpendicular penetration for 0.5 chun (1.6 cm.). Moxibustion dosage is three cones or five to ten minutes with a wick.

*Associated illnesses:* Abdominal pain, irregular menstruation, heavy menstruation, and skin rash.

45

Three points which are known to lie on the line are described here; altogether there are nine known points.

5.1 Tungli

*Site:* The point is located on the wrist, below the heel of the hand, on the side below the little finger.

*How to locate:* Seat the patient upright with his arm half bent at the elbow and the hand held with the palm up. Measure 1.0 body chun up the arm from 5.2 (Fig. 35).

*Associated treatment:* Needle depth is 0.3 chun (1 cm.). Moxibustion dosage is three cones or five to fifteen minutes with wicks.

*Associated illness:* Mental depression.

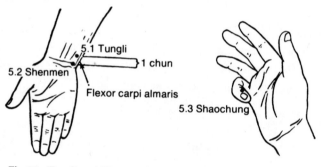

**Fig. 35**  Tungli and Shenmen          **Fig. 36**  Shaochung

5.2 Shenmen

*Site:* At the wrist wrinkle along the little-finger side near the heel of the hand.

*How to locate:* Seat the patient upright, elbow half bent, palm up. Pull and twist his little finger and ring finger outward so that a small valley appears on the little-finger side of the muscle. The point is located where this valley crosses the second wrist wrinkle (Fig. 36).

*Associated treatment:* When needling, enter at a 45-degree angle to a depth of 0.4 to 0.5 chun (1.3 to 1.6 cm.) in the direction of the little-finger side of the wrist. This depth is measured along the needle, not straight down. For moxibustion use three cones or wicks for five to fifteen minutes.

*Associated illnesses:* Insomnia, epilepsy, mental depression, and convulsions in children.

5.3 Shaochung

*Site:* The point is located along the inner side of the little finger at the base of the fingernail.

*How to locate:* Seat the patient in an upright position, palm facing downward and back of the hand facing upward. The point is at the tip of the little finger on the inner side approximately 0.1 body chun from the base of the fingernail (Fig. 36).

*Associated treatment:* Needle depth is about 0.1 chun (0.3 cm.). Moxibustion dose is three cones or five minutes with a wick.

*Associated illnesses:* Stroke and feverish illnesses. (Use this point for emergency treatment only.)


Six: Arm/Most Yang/Small Intestine

There are nineteen points along this line, three of which are considered here.

6.1 Shaotse

*Site:* The point is located on the outer side of the little finger at the base of the nail.

*How to locate:* Seat the patient in an upright position. Locate the point with the palm facing downward and the back of the hand facing upward. The point is at the tip of the little finger, approximately 0.1 body chun from the base corner of the fingernail, along the outer side of the finger (Fig. 37).

*Associated treatment:* Needle penetration depth at this point is about 0.1 chun (0.3 cm.). Moxibustion dose is three cones or heat with a wick for five minutes.

*Associated illnesses:* Stroke and feverish illness. (Use this point for emergency treatment only.)

6.2 Houshi

*Site:* The point is located above the base joint of the little finger, along the outer edge of the palm.

*How to locate:* Locate the point with the fist clenched and the fingers facing upward. The point is along the outer edge of the hand,

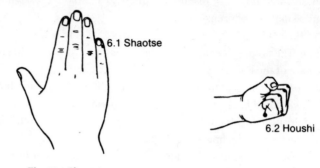

**Fig. 37**  Shaotse                    **Fig. 38**  Houshi

above the base joint of the little finger, at the terminal point of the wrinkle extending out from the palm (Fig. 38).

*Associated treatment:* Insert the needle perpendicularly to a depth of 0.3 chun (1.0 cm.). The fist should be clenched while the needle is being inserted. Moxibustion dosage is three cones or heat with a wick for five minutes.

*Associated illnesses:* Malaria, epilepsy, skin rash, and finger cramps or spasms.

6.3 Tingkung

*Site:* The point is located in the center of the cavity in front of the small ear (tragus).

*How to locate:* Seat the patient upright. Proceed along the central line of the small ear toward the front. Press down with the finger to feel a cavity. If heavy pressure produces an "uhm, uhm" sound in the ear, the point has been located (Fig. 39).

*Associated treatment:* Penetrate the needle perpendicularly to a depth of 0.3 chun (1.0 cm.). Moxibustion dosage is three cones or heat with a wick for five minutes.

*Associated illnesses:* Deafness and whistling sound in the ear.


Seven: Leg/Most Yang/Urinary Bladder

The skin line passes through sixty-seven points. We shall discuss twelve of them.

Tragus

Fig. 39  ...kung

7.1 Chingming

Site: The point is located ... the inner corner of the eye. ... it upright or lie down on his back. Measure 1.0 inch ... from ... the inner corner of the eye ... r edge of the bone at the eye ... This is the point (Fig. 40).

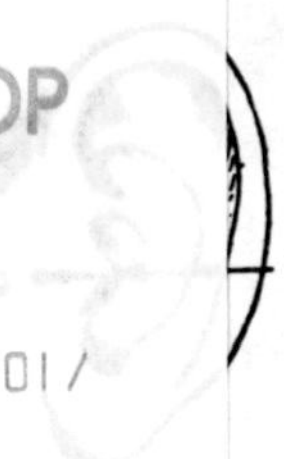

Associated treatment: Insert the ... needle to a depth of 0.1 to 0.2 chun (0.3 to 0.6 cm). Do not manipulate the needle after the insertion is completed. Leave the needle for a passive phase lasting five to fifteen minutes. Do not perform moxibustion.

Associated illnesses: Soreness of the eyes and windburned eyes.

7.2 Tsanchu

Site: The point is located in the center of the cavity near the peak of the eyebrow.

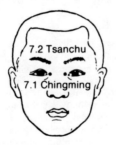

**Fig. 40**  Chingming and Tsanchu

49

*How to locate:* Let the patient sit upright. Measure toward the middle from the peak of the eyebrow along the brow for 1.0 body chun. This is the location of the point (Fig. 40).

*Associated treatment:* Penetrate the needle at the edge of the eyebrow with the needle parallel to the skin, moving sideways toward the nose for a distance of about 0.1 chun (0.3 cm.). Moxibustion is not applicable at this point.

*Associated illnesses:* Aching eyebrow bone, windburned eyes, and soreness of the eyes.

### 7.3 Tachu

*Site:* The points are located at the two sides below the first spinal bone unit on the back.

*How to locate:* Seat the patient in an upright position. Feel with the hand from the back of the neck along the spinal column downward. After finding the highest protruding spinal column bone at the base of the neck (the seventh atlas), feel below this bone for the first back spinal bone (the first thoracic vertebra). At the base cavity of this bone, measure 1.5 body chuns sideways on each side. These are the points.[1]

*Associated treatment:* Penetrate the needle perpendicularly to a depth of 0.3 to 0.5 chun (1.0 to 1.6 cm.). Moxibustion dosage is three to seven cones or ten to twenty minutes with a wick.

*Associated illnesses:* Coughing, toothache, and headache at the top of the head.

### 7.4 Feishu

*Site:* On the two sides of the spine below the third vertebra.

---

1. In acupuncture terms, the human spinal column consists of twenty-one bone units—the first vertebra through the twenty-first. The corresponding anatomical designations are as follows: the first twelve vertebrae are the twelve thoracic vertebrae of the rib cage; the thirteenth to the seventeenth are the five lumbar vertebrae at the waist; the eighteenth to the twenty-first vertebrae are the four coccygeal vertebrae. In this book we use the acupuncture numbering of the vertebrae. Points will be located by counting the vertebrae from the first bone (the top bone) downward and then moving to either side for an indicated number of body chuns.

*How to locate:* Seat the patient upright or have the patient lie prone. Along either duct below the third vertebra, measure sideways away from the spine 1.5 body chuns. This is the point (Fig. 41).

*Associated treatment:* Penetrate the needle perpendicularly to a depth of 0.3 to 0.5 chun (1.0 to 1.6 cm.). Moxibustion dosage is five to seven cones, or five to twenty minutes with the wicks.

*Associated illnesses:* Coughing and whooping cough.

7.5 Keshu

*Site:* The point is located on the two sides of the spine, below the seventh vertebra.

*How to locate:* Have the patient sit upright or lie prone. Measure sideways along either duct below the seventh vertebra (the seventh thoracic vertebra) for a distance of 1.5 body chuns from the spine. This is the point (Fig. 41).

*Associated treatment:* Penetrate the needle to a depth of 0.3 to 0.5 chun (1.0 to 1.6 cm.). Moxibustion dosage is five cones or five to ten minutes with a wick.

*Associated illnesses:* Belching, failure to menstruate, chest pains, and bloody stools.

7.6 Pishu

*Site:* On either side of the spine below the eleventh vertebra.

*How to locate:* Have the patient sit upright or lie prone. Measure sideways along either duct below the eleventh vertebra (the eleventh thoracic vertebra) for 1.5 body chuns away from the spine. This is the point (Fig. 41).

*Associated treatment:* Penetrate the needle to a depth of 0.3 to 0.5 chun (1.0 to 1.6 cm.). Moxibustion dosage is three cones or five to ten minutes with a wick.

*Associated illnesses:* Indigestion, vomiting, diarrhea, and ir-regular menstruation.

7.7 Weishu

*Site:* On either side of the spine below the twelfth vertebra.

*How to locate:* Have the patient sit upright or lie prone. Measure sideways along either duct below the twelfth vertebra (the twelfth cervical vertebra) for 1.5 body chuns away from the spine. This is the point (Fig. 41).

*Associated treatment:* Penetrate the needle perpendicularly to a depth of 0.3 to 0.5 chun (1.0 to 1.6 cm.). Moxibustion dosage is five cones or five to twenty minutes with the wicks.

*Associated illnesses:* Intestinal noises, indigestion or heartburn, vomiting, and diarrhea.

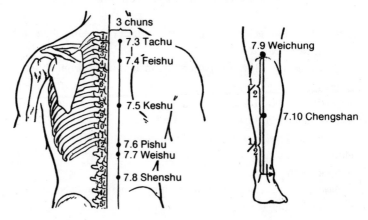

**Fig. 41** Tachu, Feishu, Keshu, Pishu, Weishu, and Shenshu

**Fig. 42** Weichung and Chengshan

7.8 Shenshu

*Site:* Along either side of the spine below the fourteenth vertebra.

*How to locate:* Have the patient sit upright or lie prone. Measure sideways along either duct below the fourteenth vertebra (the second lumbar vertebra) for 1.5 body chuns from the spine. This is the point (Fig. 41).

*Associated treatment:* Penetrate the needle to a depth of 0.5 to 0.8 chun (1.6 to 2.6 cm.). Moxibustion dosage is five cones or five to twenty minutes with the wicks.

*Associated illnesses:* Waist or back (spinal) pain, early-morning diarrhea, bed-wetting, irregular menstruation, painful menstruation, failure to menstruate, and bloody stools.

### 7.9 Weichung

*Site:* On the back of the knee, at the center of the curve as the knee bends.

*How to locate:* Have the patient lie down in the prone position. The point is located at the midpoint of the wrinkle crossing the cavity at the back of the knee (Fig. 42).

*Associated treatment:* Penetrate the needle to a depth of 0.5 to 1.0 chun (1.6 to 3.2 cm.). An aching and swelling sensation may reach as far up as the hip and as far down as the toes. A trocar needle may also be used to let blood at this point. Do not administer moxibustion.

*Associated illnesses:* Aching at the back of the waist, abdominal pain, knee aches, fever, thirst, cramps or spasms of the arms or legs, boils or carbuncles, appendicitis pain, skin rash, and heatstroke.

### 7.10 Chengshan

*Site:* On the back of the calf.

*How to locate:* Have the patient standing up and tiptoed forward. A ⋏ shape formation will appear at the lower part of the muscular bulge of the leg; the point is located at the apex of the formation (7.0 body chuns vertically down from 7.9). If the ⋏ shape is vague and ambiguous, locate the point by locating the midpoint of the line joining 7.9 and the tip of the back protrusion of the heel bone (Fig. 43).

*Associated treatment:* Penetrate the needle to a depth of 0.7 chun (2.2 cm.). Moxibustion dosage is three to five cones or five to fifteen minutes with the wicks.

*Associated illnesses:* Aches in the arms or the legs, leg cramps, and constipation.

### 7.11 Kunlun

*Site:* At the center of the cavity behind the outer ankle bulge.

*How to locate:* Have the patient sitting upright, and place his foot flat (on a support). Apply finger pressure to locate a cavity approximately 0.5 body chun behind the outer ankle. On the front side of the cavity is the ankle bone, on the back side is the ankle tendon (tendo calcan) and below it is the heel bone. The point is located

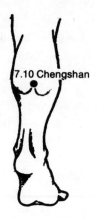

**Fig. 43**   Chengshan

between the tip of the ankle bone and the tendon (Fig. 44). This point is situated in symmetry with 8.2 (on the kidney skin line).

*Associated treatment:* Penetrate the needle perpendicularly to a depth of 0.5 chun (1.6 cm.). Needle treatment is forbidden if the patient is pregnant. Moxibustion dosage is three cones or five to ten minutes with a wick.

*Associated illnesses:* Headache, aching at the back of the waist, sprained foot, leg cramps or spasms, backward arching of the body, leg paralysis, convulsions in children, and difficult childbirth.

7.12 Chihyin

*Site:* The point is located at the outer edge of the little toe, at the base of the nail.

*How to locate:* Have the patient's foot placed flat. At the outer edge of the little (fifth) toe, locate the point at 0.1 body chun from the base corner of the nail (Fig. 44).

*Associated treatment:* Penetrate the needle at a 45-degree insertion angle. Moxibustion dosage is three to five cones or five minutes with a wick.

*Associated illnesses:* Insomnia and difficult childbirth.

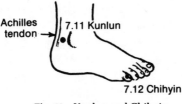

**Fig. 44**  Kunlun and Chihyin

EIGHT: LEG/LEAST YIN/KIDNEY

Twenty-seven acupuncture points are known on this line. We shall consider three of them.

8.1 Yungchuan

*Site:* On the front half of the sole, along the central line.

*How to locate:* Locate the point with the patient lying supine. Have the patient curl the five toes downward; a cavity will show at the central region of the upper sole. This is the point (Fig. 45).

*Associated treatment:* Penetrate the needle perpendicularly to a depth of 0.3 to 0.5 chun (1.0 to 1.6 cm.). Moxibustion dosage is three cones or five to fifteen minutes with the wicks.

*Associated illnesses:* Headache at the sides, stupor and continuous unconsciousness, and epilepsy.

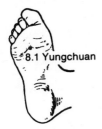

**Fig. 45**  Yungchuan

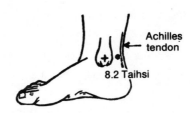

**Fig. 46**  Taihsi

55

8.2 Taihsi

*Site:* At the center of the cavity situated behind the inner ankle.

*How to locate:* Seat the patient upright, with his foot flat and propped up, or have the patient lie supine. Measure 0.5 body chun from the inner ankle backward. Apply finger pressure to locate a cavity. On one side of this cavity is the ankle bone; on the other side is a tendon (tendo calcan), and below the cavity is the heel bone. The point is located between the tip of the ankle bone and the tendon (Fig. 46). This point is in symmetry with 7.11 (on the urinary bladder skin line).

*Associated treatment:* Penetrate the needle perpendicularly to a depth of 0.3 to 0.5 chun (1.0 to 1.6 cm.). Moxibustion dosage is three to seven cones or five to ten minutes with a wick.

*Associated illnesses:* Sprained foot, dizziness and nausea, toothache, and belching.

8.3 Chaohai

*Site:* Below the inner ankle.

*How to locate:* Have the patient seated firmly, and close his feet together, sole to sole. Proceeding from the sharp point of the inner ankle downward in the direction of the sole, the point is located at the crevice at the base of the ankle (Fig. 47).

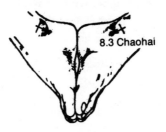

**Fig. 47**   Chaohai

*Associated treatment:* Penetrate the needle perpendicularly to a depth of 0.3 to 0.5 chun (1.0 to 1.6 cm.). Moxibustion dosage is three to seven cones or five to ten minutes with a wick.

*Associated illnesses:* Constipation and early-morning diarrhea.

There are nine known points located on this skin line. We describe four of them.

9.1 Chutse

*Site:* At the center of the elbow cavity.

*How to locate:* Locate the point with the patient's arm stretched out, palm up. Along the longitudinal wrinkle crossing the elbow cavity, feel for a large tendon (tendon of brachioradialis). Locate the point on the inner (ulnar) side of this tendon (Fig. 48).

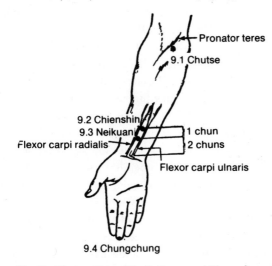

**Fig. 48**   Chutse, Chienshih, Neikuan, and Chungchung

*Associated treatment:* Penetrate the needle perpendicularly to a depth of 0.3 chun (1.0 cm.). Moxibustion dosage is three cones or five to ten minutes with a wick.

*Associated illnesses:* Cramps and spasms in the arms or legs, appendicitis pain, and vomiting.

9.2 Chienshih

*Site:* On the forearm, along the central line of the inner surface, 3.0 body chuns up the arm from the bend of the wrist.

*How to locate:* Have the patient clench his fist, palm up. From the midpoint of the wrist wrinkle at the base of the palm, measure up the forearm for a distance of 3.0 body chuns. Locate the point between the two longitudinal tendons (flexor carpi umaris and flexor carpi radialis) (Fig. 48).

*Associated treatment:* Penetrate the needle perpendicularly to a depth of 0.3 to 0.5 chun (1.0 to 1.6 cm.). Moxibustion dosage is three cones or five to ten minutes with a wick.

*Associated illnesses:* Malaria, epilepsy, and chest or rib pains.

9.3 Neikuan

*Site:* Along the central line on the inner side of the forearm, 2.0 body chuns up from the bend of the wrist.

*How to locate:* Locate the point with the patient's fist clenched, palm up. From the midpoint of the first wrinkle at the base of the palm, proceed upward along the arm for 2.0 body chuns. Here locate the point between the two longitudinal tendons (Fig. 48).

*Associated treatment:* Penetrate the needle perpendicularly to a depth of 0.3 to 0.5 chun (1.0 to 1.6 cm.). An aching and swelling sensation sometimes reaches up to the elbow area, the shoulder, the neck, or even to the ear. In the other direction the sensation reaches as far as the middle finger. Moxibustion dosage at this point is three to five cones or five to ten minutes with a wick.

*Associated illnesses:* Indigestion or heartburn, vomiting, chest or rib pains, belching, insomnia, cholera, heatstroke, abdominal pain, mental depression, discomfort in the chest, and convulsions in children.

9.4 Chungchung

*Site:* At the tip of the middle finger.

*How to locate:* Locate the point with the hand stretched, palm up. The point is at the tip of the middle finger, approximately at a distance of 0.1 body chun from the fingernail (Fig. 48).

*Associated treatment:* Penetrate the needle to a depth of 0.1 chun (0.3 cm.). Moxibustion dosage is one cone or five minutes with a wick.

*Associated illnesses:* Convulsions in children and unconsciousness. (For emergency treatment.)

There are twenty-three known points located on this skin line. We choose seven of them.

10.1 Kuanchung

*Site:* At the outer edge (the side adjacent to the little finger) of the ring finger (the fourth finger), near the base of the fingernail.

*How to locate:* Locate the point with the patient's hand stretched, palm down. The point is along the outer edge of the fourth finger, at a distance of 0.1 body chun from the base corner of the fingernail (Fig. 49).

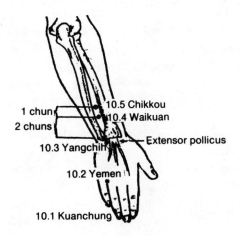

**Fig. 49** Kuanchung, Yemen, Yangchih, Waikuan, and Chihkou

*Associated treatment:* Penetrate the needle at a 45-degree angle to a depth of 0.1 chun (0.3 cm.). Moxibustion dosage is three cones or five minutes with a wick.

*Associated illnesses:* Unconsciousness. (For emergency treatment.)

10.2 Yemen

*Site:* Near the end of the valley between the ring finger and the little finger (the fourth and fifth fingers).

*How to locate:* Locate the point with the patient's hand stretched, palm down. Find the point at a short distance behind the apex of the cleavage between the ring and the little fingers (Fig. 49).

*Associated treatment:* With the needle, use perpendicular insertion to a depth of 0.3 chun (1.0 cm.). Moxibustion dosage is three cones or about five minutes with a wick.

*Associated illnesses:* Pain at the back of the hand, insufficient mother's milk, headache, and malaria.

10.3 Yangchih

*Site:* On the back (dorsal surface) of the wrist near the center.

*How to locate:* Locate the point with the patient's hand outstretched, palm down, elbow half bent. On the outer side of the wrist a large central tendon (flexor) crosses the joint area of the carpus (ring-finger bone). The point is found at the cavity on the ulnar (little-finger) side of this tendon (Fig. 49).

*Associated treatment:* Penetrate the needle perpendicularly to a depth of 0.5 chun (1.6 cm.). Do not administer moxibustion at this point.

*Associated illnesses:* Wrist pains and headache.

10.4 Waikuan

*Site:* On the back (dorsal surface) of the forearm, 2.0 body chuns up from the wrist between the bones.

*How to locate:* Raise the patient's arm to the horizontal position, half bent at the elbow, palm down. From 10.3, measure 2.0 body chuns upward along the valley between the two arm bones (ulna and radius). This is the point (Fig. 49). This point is in symmetry with 9.3 (on the pericardium skin line).

*Associated treatment:* Penetrate the needle to a depth of 0.3 to 0.6 chun (1.0 to 1.9 cm.). Aching and swelling sensations sometimes reach up to the elbow, and sometimes as far as the shoulder or the neck. The sensation reaches down as far as the fingers. Moxibustion dosage is three cones or five to ten minutes with a wick.

*Associated illnesses:* Headache, toothache, chest or rib pains, pain in the elbow, deafness, continuous unconsciousness or stupor, mumps, and constipation after childbirth.

10.5 Chihkou

*Site:* On the back (dorsal surface) of the forearm, 3.0 body chuns from the bend of the wrist.

*How to locate:* Raise the patient's arm to the horizontal position, elbow half bent, palm down. Measure 1.0 body chun up from 10.4 along the valley between the two arm bones. This is the point (Fig. 49). This point is in symmetry with 9.2 (on the pericardium skin line).

*Associated treatment:* Penetrate the needle perpendicularly to a depth of 0.3 to 0.6 chun (1.0 to 1.9 cm.). Moxibustion dosage is three cones or five to ten minutes with a wick.

*Associated illnesses:* Chest or rib pains, indigestion or heartburn, wrist pain, constipation, vomiting, and aftereffects of childbirth.

10.6 Yifeng

*Site:* The point is located at the cavity on the upper part of the neck behind the earlobe.

*How to locate:* Seat the patient upright. Behind the earlobe, at a distance of 0.5 body chun from the end point of the lobe contour, feel with finger pressure for a cavity. The point is reached when the patient feels tense and uncomfortable as a result of the pressure (Fig. 50).

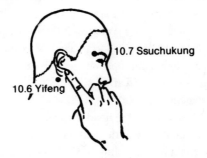

**Fig. 50**  Yifeng and Ssuchukung

*Associated treatment:* Penetrate the needle perpendicularly to a depth of 0.3 to 0.5 chun (1.0 to 1.6 cm.). Moxibustion dosage is three cones or five to ten minutes with a wick.

*Associated illnesses:* Whistling noise in the ear, deafness, and mumps.

10.7 Ssuchukung

*Site:* At the lateral end-point of the brow.

*How to locate:* Seat the patient upright. At the lateral end of the brow there is a cavity. This is the point (Fig. 50).

*Associated treatment:* Penetrate the needle with the tip toward the midpoint of the brow and the needle parallel to the skin. Penetrate to a depth of 0.3 to 0.5 chun (1.0 to 1.6 cm.). Do not administer moxibustion at this point.

*Associated illnesses:* Headache on the sides, redness and soreness of the eye, and pains at the brow (frontal) bone.


ELEVEN: LEG/LEAST YANG/GALLBLADDER

There are forty-four known points on this skin line. We describe six points.

11.1 Tinghui

*Site:* In front of the ear, near the lower end of tragus.

*How to locate:* Seat the patient upright. At the merging line of the ear and the face, on the level of the antetragus, feel with the hand for a cavity as the patient opens his mouth. This is the point (Fig. 51).

*Associated treatment:* Penetrate the needle perpendicularly to a depth of 0.2 to 0.3 chun (0.6 to 1.0 cm.). Moxibustion dosage is three cones or five to ten minutes with a wick.

*Associated illness:* Deafness.

11.2 Fengchih

*Site:* On the back of the head at the neck.

*How to locate:* Seat the patient upright, head bent forward. Proceed from the center line of the back of the neck upward for a distance of 1.0 body chun beyond the hairline, then move sideways toward the ear for a distance of 1.5 body chuns. At this point there is a cavity between two neck muscles and above the hairline. This is the point (Fig. 52).

*Associated treatment:* Penetrate the needle to a depth of 0.5 to 0.8 chun (1.6 to 2.6 cm.). When applying the needle to the left point, the

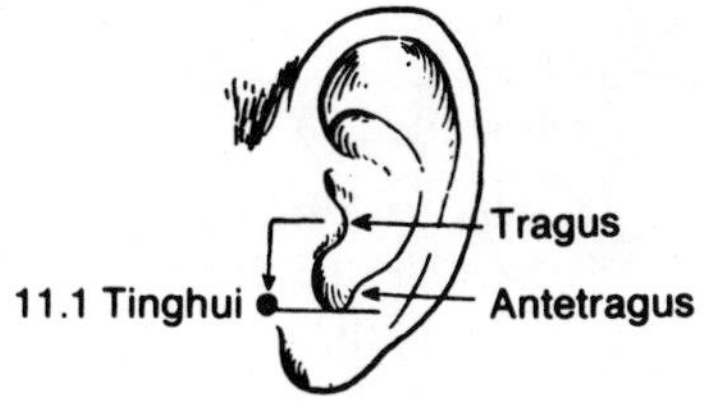

**Fig. 51**  Tinghui

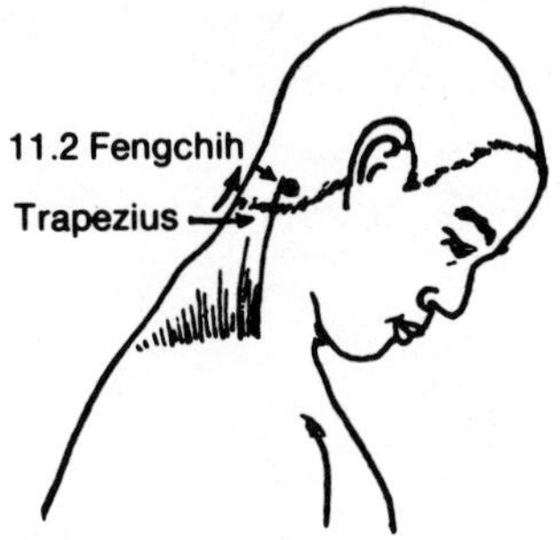

**Fig. 52**  Fengchih

tip of the needle should point toward the right eye; it should point toward the left eye when the needle is applied to the right point. An aching and swelling sensation may reach upward to the top of the head and to the eye socket; downward the sensation reaches as far as the end of the shoulder. Moxibustion dosage is three cones or five to fifteen minutes with the wicks.

*Associated illnesses:* Headache, colds and influenza, fever, coughing, mumps, convulsions in children, toothache, windburned eyes, and whooping cough.

11.3 Hsuantiao

*Site:* On the side of the hip.

*How to locate:* Have the patient lying on one side or squatting. Locate the tip of the tailbone (coccyx), and measure upward for a distance of two finger widths. Then measure horizontally sideways along either side, over the large hip muscle bulge toward the pointed edge of the hipbone (ilium). Divide this line into three equal parts. The point is located in the cavity one-third of the distance from the tip of the hipbone (Fig. 53).

*Associated treatment:* Penetrate the needle perpendicularly to a depth of 0.2 to 0.3 chun (0.6 to 1.0 cm.). Frequently the aching and swelling sensation moves along the back side of the thigh down toward the toes. Moxibustion dosage is seven cones or ten to twenty minutes with the wicks.

*Associated illnesses:* Pains in the waist or legs, paralysis of half the body, and pains in the leg due to damp surroundings (arthritic or rheumatic pains).

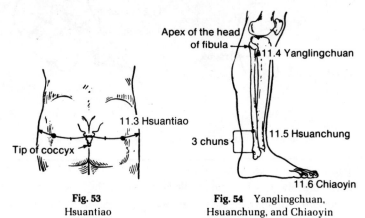

**Fig. 53**
Hsuantiao

**Fig. 54**  Yanglingchuan,
Hsuanchung, and Chiaoyin

11.4 Yanglingchuan

*Site:* Below the knee on the lateral side.

*How to locate:* Seat the patient upright with the knees bent and feet dangling, or have the patient lie down, legs stretched. At the lateral side of the knee, feel for a round bone protrusion (tip of the fibula) below the knee. Below this round protrusion is a cavity. This is the point (Fig. 54).

*Associated treatment:* Penetrate the needle perpendicularly to a depth of 0.8 to 1.2 chuns (2.6 to 3.8 cm.). An aching sensation sometimes reaches down toward the third and the fourth toe. Upward the sensation sometimes reaches the rib area under the arm. Moxibustion dosage is three cones or five to ten minutes with a wick.

*Associated illnesses:* Paralysis of the legs, pain at the knee, headache, failure to urinate, and bending and twisting of the extremities.

11.5 Hsuanchung

*Site:* 3.0 body chuns above the lateral tip of the ankle.

*How to locate:* Seat the patient upright, feet dangling. From the lateral tip of the ankle, measure upward along the fibula. This is the point (Fig. 54).

*Associated treatment:* Penetrate the needle perpendicularly to a depth of 0.3 to 0.5 chun (1.0 to 1.6 cm.). Moxibustion dosage is three to five cones or five to ten minutes with the wicks.

*Associated illnesses:* Headache at the sides, paralysis of half the body, crick in the neck, and pain at the knee or ankle.

11.6 Chiaoyin

*Site:* On the fourth toe, at the side adjacent to the little toe, near the base corner of the nail.

*How to locate:* Seat the patient upright. The point is on the fourth toe, along the edge adjacent to the little toe, at a distance of 0.1 body chun from the base corner of the nail (Fig. 54).

*Associated treatment:* Penetrate the needle to a depth of 0.1 chun (0.3 cm.). Moxibustion dosage is three cones or five minutes with a wick.

*Associated illnesses:* Headache and chest or rib pains.


TWELVE: LEG/NORMAL YIN/LIVER

There are fourteen known points on this skin line. We choose three points.

12.1 Tatun

*Site:* On the upper side of the toe, near the base of the nail.

*How to locate:* Have the patient lie supine or sit upright. From the midpoint of the base of the toenail, proceed upward 0.1 body chun, then measure sideways 0.1 body chun in the direction of the little toe. This is the point (Fig. 55).

*Associated treatment:* Penetrate the needle at a 45-degree angle to a depth of 0.1 to 0.2 chun (0.3 to 0.6 cm.). Moxibustion dosage is three cones or three to five minutes with a wick.

*Associated illnesses:* Heavy menstruation and bed-wetting.

12.2 Hsingchien

*Site:* At the end of the valley between the first and second toes (Fig. 55).

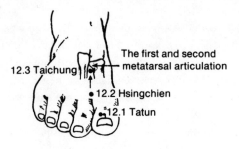

**Fig. 55** Tatun, Hsingchien, and Taichung

*Associated treatment:* Penetrate the needle to a depth of 0.3 chun (1.0 cm.). Moxibustion dosage is three cones or five to ten minutes with a wick.

*Associated illnesses:* Toothache, irregular menstruation, and failure to menstruate.

12.3 Taichung

*Site:* In front of the angle between the first and second toe bones (metatarsals) on the upper face of the foot.

*How to locate:* Have the patient lie supine or sit upright. From the end of the valley between the first and second toes, push upward with index finger along the valley for 2.0 body chuns until a cavity in front of the joint (fossa of the first and second metatarsals) is reached. This is the point (Fig. 55).

*Associated treatment:* Penetrate the needle perpendicularly to a depth of 0.3 chun (1.0 cm.). Moxibustion dosage is three cones or five minutes with a wick.

*Associated illnesses:* Headache, sore throat, chest or rib pains, pains of the feet, pinkeye, and irregular menstruation.

THIRTEEN: JEN VESSEL (VESSEL OF CONCEPTION)

Twenty points are known to lie along this line, seven of which are within the scope of this book.

13.1 Chungchi

*Site:* Below the navel.

*How to locate:* Have the patient lie supine. The point is located on the midline, 4.0 body chuns below the navel (Fig. 56).

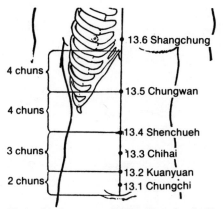

**Fig. 56**   Chungchi, Kuanyuan, Chihai, Shenchueh, Chungwan, and Shanchung

*Associated treatment:* Penetrate the needle to a depth of 0.8 to 1.0 chun (2.6 to 3.2 cm.). Needle treatment is forbidden if the patient is pregnant. Moxibustion dosage is five cones or five to fifteen minutes with the wicks.

*Associated illnesses:* Bed-wetting, irregular menstruation, heavy menstruation, and failure to menstruate.

13.2 Kuanyuan

*Site:* Below the navel.

*How to locate:* Have the patient lie supine. The point is located 3.0 body chuns directly below the navel, 1.0 body chun above 13.1 (Fig. 56).

*Associated treatment:* Penetrate the needle perpendicularly to a depth of 0.8 to 1.5 chuns (2.6 to 4.8 cm.). Needle treatment is forbidden at this point if the patient is pregnant. Moxibustion dosage is seven cones or five to fifteen minutes with the wicks.

*Associated illnesses:* Backache at the waist, pain around the navel, bed-wetting, irregular menstruation, heavy menstruation, painful menstruation, aftereffects of childbirth, apoplexy or loose strokes, and appendix pain.

13.3 Chihai

*Site:* Below the navel.

*How to locate:* Have the patient lie supine. The point is located 1.5 body chuns directly below the navel (Fig. 56).

*Associated treatment:* Penetrate the needle perpendicularly to a depth of 0.8 to 1.5 chuns (2.6 to 4.8 cm.). Needle treatment is forbidden if the patient is pregnant. Moxibustion dosage is seven cones or five to fifteen minutes with the wicks.

*Associated illnesses:* Abdominal pain, early-morning diarrhea, backache at the waist, bed-wetting, irregular menstruation, heavy menstruation, painful menstruation, failure to menstruate, aftereffects of childbirth, and apoplexy or loose strokes.

13.4 Shenchueh

*Site:* At the center of the navel.

*How to locate:* Have the patient lie supine. The point is at the center of the navel (Fig. 56).

*Associated treatment:* Moxibustion dosage may vary from five to fifteen or to several dozen cones, all over salt. Do not administer needle treatment at this point.

*Associated illnesses:* Intestinal pain and noises, diarrhea, dysentery, apoplexy or loose strokes, aftereffects of childbirth, and baby's lockjaw (from unhygienic cutting of the umbilical cord).

13.5 Chungwan

*Site:* On the midline 4.0 body chuns above the navel.

*How to locate:* Have the patient lie supine. The point is 4.0 body chuns directly above the navel, which is also half of the distance from the navel to the chest cavity (Fig. 56).

*Associated treatment:* Penetrate perpendicularly to a depth of 0.8 to 1.0 chun (2.6 to 3.2 cm.). Moxibustion dosage is seven cones or five to fifteen minutes with the wicks.

*Associated illnesses:* Indigestion or heartburn, pressure and swelling in the abdomen, vomiting acid, diarrhea, dysentery, constipation, and cholera.

### 13.6 Shanchung

*Site:* On the chest between the nipples or breasts.

*How to locate:* Have the patient lie supine. The point is located on the central dividing line of the chest, halfway between the breast nipples (Fig. 56).

*Associated treatment:* Penetrate with the needle parallel to the skin with the tip directed downward to a depth of 0.3 to 0.5 chun (1.0 to 1.6 cm.). Moxibustion dosage is five cones or five to fifteen minutes with the wicks.

*Associated illness:* Insufficient mother's milk.

### 13.7 Chengchiang

*Site:* Beneath the lower lip.

*How to locate:* Have the patient open his mouth. The point is located along the central line dividing the lips and the chin, inside the cavity beneath the lower lip (Fig. 57).

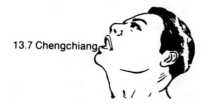

13.7 Chengchiang

**Fig. 57** Chengchiang

*Associated treatment:* Penetrate perpendicularly to a depth of 0.3 chun (1.0 cm.). Moxibustion dosage is one cone or five minutes with a wick.

*Associated illnesses:* Stiff neck and epilepsy.

### FOURTEEN: TU VESSEL (GOVERNING VESSEL)

Twenty-eight points are known along this vessel, eleven of which are described here.

### 14.1 Changchiang

*Site:* Between the tip of the tailbone and the anus.

*How to locate:* The patient assumes a squatting position, with the upper body leaning forward. This point is located in the cavity situated between the tip of the tailbone and the anus (Fig. 58).

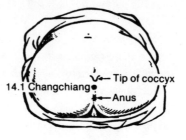

**Fig. 58**   Changchiang

*Associated treatment:* Penetrate perpendicularly to a depth of 0.5 to 1.0 chun (1.6 to 3.2 cm.). Moxibustion dosage is three cones or five minutes with a wick.

*Associated illnesses:* Protrusion of the end of the colon at the anus and bloody stools.

14.2 Yaoshu

*Site:* Inside the cavity below the twenty-first vertebra.

*How to locate:* The patient assumes a squatting position, leaning forward. The point is in the cavity below the twenty-first vertebra (between the fourth sacral vertebra and the coccyx) (Fig. 59).

*Associated treatment:* Penetrate perpendicularly to a depth of 0.3 to 0.5 chun (1.0 to 1.6 cm.). Moxibustion dosage is seven cones or five to fifteen minutes with the wicks.

*Associated illness:* Backache.

14.3 Mingmen

*Site:* Inside the cavity situated below the fourteenth vertebra.

*How to locate:* The patient sits upright or squats with the upper body leaning forward. The point is at the center of the cavity below the fourteenth vertebra (the second lumbar vertebra) (Fig. 59). This point is in matching symmetry with the navel (13.4 of the Jen vessel) (Fig. 60).

*Associated treatment:* Penetrate perpendicularly to a depth of 0.3 to 0.5 chun (1.0 to 1.6 cm.). Moxibustion dosage is three cones or five to fifteen minutes with the wicks.

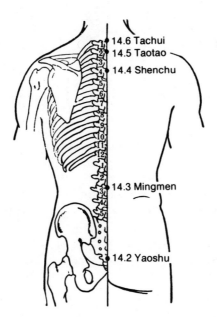

**Fig. 59**   Yaoshu, Mingmen, Shenchu, Taotao, and Tachui

*Associated illnesses:* Pain at the back of the waist, abdominal pain, irregular menstruation, painful menstruation, heavy menstruation, and bloody stools.

14.4 Shenchu

*Site:* Inside the cavity below the third (thoracic) vertebra.

*How to locate:* The patient sits upright or squats. Locate the cavity below the third (thoracic) vertebra. The point is at the center of the cavity (Fig. 59).

*Associated treatment:* Penetrate upward at a 45-degree angle to a depth of 0.3 to 0.5 chun (1.0 to 1.6 cm.). Moxibustion dosage is three to five cones or five to ten minutes with a wick.

*Associated illnesses:* Pains in the back or at the waist and boils or carbuncles.

14.5 Taotao

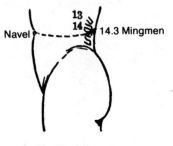

**Fig. 60**   Mingmen

*Site:* Inside the cavity below the first vertebra.

*How to locate:* Have the patient sit upright with his head bent forward. Locate the cavity below the first vertebra (the first thoracic vertebra). The point is at the center of the cavity (Fig. 59).

*Associated treatment:* Penetrate perpendicularly to a depth of 0.3 to 0.8 chun (1.0 to 2.6 cm.). Moxibustion dosage is five cones or five minutes with a wick.

*Associated illnesses:* Malaria and fever.

14.6 Tachui

*Site:* Inside the cavity above the first vertebra.

*How to locate:* Have the patient sit upright, head leaning forward. Locate the cavity above the first vertebra (between the seventh cervical vertebra and the first thoracic vertebra). The point is at the center of the cavity (Fig. 59).

*Associated treatment:* Penetrate perpendicularly to a depth of 0.5 chun (1.6 cm.). Moxibustion dosage is five to seven cones or five to fifteen minutes with the wicks.

*Associated illnesses:* Colds or influenza, fever, vomiting, malaria, stiff neck, convulsions in children, epilepsy, crick in the neck, toothache, pinkeye, whooping cough, and coughing.

14.7 Yamen

*Site:* Along the middle line of the back of the neck, inside the hairline.

*How to locate:* Have the patient sit upright, head bent forward.

Proceed upward along the midline of the back of the neck; at a distance of 0.5 body chun from the hairline (between the first and the second cervical vertebrae). This is the point (Fig. 61).

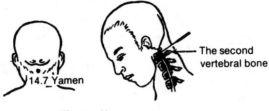

**Fig. 61**    Yamen

*Associated treatment:* For elderly or thin patients, penetration depth should be about 1.5 chuns (4.8 cm.). For heavier patients, penetrate to about 2.0 chuns (6.4 cm.). When administering acupuncture at this point, greatest care must be given to the angle of penetration. The needle should be angled downward in the direction of the throat of the patient. *Under no circumstance may the needle be penetrated upward.* The needle should be inserted slowly, without any side motion. If at any time the patient feels a sensation resembling electric shock, the needle must be extracted immediately. After penetrating to a depth of about 2.0 chuns (6.4 cm.), if the patient feels no sensation and does not react, do not penetrate farther; this is to prevent accidents.

*Associated illness:* Deafness.

14.8 Paihui

*Site:* On the top of the head.

*How to locate:* Have the patient sit upright or sit supported with the head leaning backward. The point is on the top of the head. Begin at the point 1.0 body chun above the brow level on the midline of the face; proceed along this midline toward the hairline at the back side of the neck. The acupuncture point is located midway along this line (Figs. 62 and 63).

*Associated treatment:* Penetrate the needle (almost) parallel to the skin; direct the needle tip toward the back side of the head to a

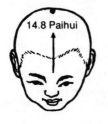

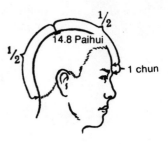

**Fig. 62**  Paihui            **Fig. 63**  Paihui

depth of 0.2 to 0.3 chun (0.6 to 1.0 cm.). Moxibustion dosage is three cones or five to seven minutes with a wick.

*Associated illnesses:* Apoplexy or strokes, headache, dizziness or nausea, epilepsy, protrusion of the bowel, fever, stiff neck, nosebleed, deafness and dumbness, and diarrhea in children.

14.9 Shanghsing

*Site:* On the forehead, 1.0 body chun above the hairline.

*How to locate:* Have the patient sit upright or lie supine. Proceed upward from the midpoint between the two brow ends to reach the hairline and 1.0 body chun beyond. This is the point (Fig. 64).

*Associated treatment:* Penetrate with the needle parallel to the skin and the tip directed toward the top of the head to a depth of 0.2 to 0.3 chun (0.6 to 1.0 cm.). Moxibustion dosage is three cones or five minutes with a wick.

*Associated illnesses:* Headache, sinus congestion, and nosebleed.

14.10 Shenting

*Site:* On the middle of the forehead, 0.5 body chun above the hairline.

*How to locate:* Have the patient sit upright or lie supine. Proceed upward from the midpoint between the two brow ends to reach the hairline. Locate the point at 0.5 chun more into the hairline (Fig. 64).

*Associated treatment:* Penetrate with the needle parallel to the skin, directing the tip toward the top of the head. Penetrate to a depth of 0.2 to 0.3 chun (0.6 to 1.0 cm.). Moxibustion dosage is three cones or five minutes with a wick.

*Associated illnesses:* Headache, pains at the brow ridges, and epilepsy.

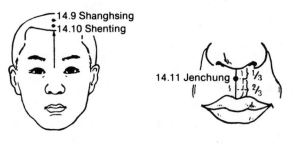

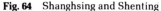

**Fig. 64**   Shanghsing and Shenting

**Fig. 65**   Jenchung

14.11 Jenchung (or Waterduct)

*Site:* At the middle of the duct below the nose.

*How to locate:* Have the patient sit upright with support at the back of the head, the head leaning backward, or lay him supine. The point is located on the valley of the upper lip (called the waterduct), one-third of its length from the nose (Fig. 65).

*Associated treatment:* Penetrate, with the tip of the needle directed slightly upward or downward, to a depth of 0.2 to 0.3 chun (0.6 to 1.0 cm.). Remove the needle as soon as pain is felt; thus, it is not necessary to leave the needle for a passive phase. Do not administer moxibustion at this point.

*Associated illnesses:* Epilepsy, tightly clenched teeth, apoplexy or strokes (the loose type), unconsciousness or stupor, cramps or spasms of the extremities, and convulsions in children. This is the point at which emergency reviving treatment for sudden fainting is administered.

FIFTEEN: THE ISOLATED BODY POINTS

We shall discuss thirteen such points.

15.1 Yintang

*Site:* Between the brow ends (on the nose ridge).

*How to locate:* Seat the patient upright and support the neck, head leaning backward, or lay him supine. The point is in the cavity on the nose ridge, centered between the two eyebrows, in line with the nose tip (Fig. 66).

*Associated treatment:* With the needle almost parallel to the skin, penetrate upward or downward to a distance of 0.1 or 0.2 chun (0.3 to 0.6 cm.). Do not administer moxibustion at this point.

*Associated illnesses:* Headache, and convulsions in children.

15.2 Taiyang

*Site:* On the lateral side of the face, near the corner of the eye, a short distance above the eye level.

*How to locate:* Have the patient sit upright or lean back on a support, head up. From the point between the brow end and the eye corner, measure backward 1.0 body chun, feel and locate a cavity. This is the point (Fig. 66).

*Associated treatment:* Penetrate to a depth of 0.3 to 0.5 chun (1.0 to 1.6 cm.). This point may also be stabbed to let blood.

*Associated illnesses:* Headache on the sides and pinkeye.

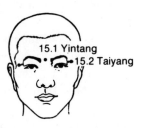 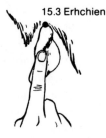

**Fig. 66**   Yintang and Taiyang        **Fig. 67**   Erhchien

15.3 Erhchien

*Site:* On the upper tip of the ear.

*How to locate:* Seat the patient upright. Bend the ear forward. The point is at the upper tip of the ear (the helix) (Fig. 67).

*Associated treatment:* Stab this point to let blood.

*Associated illnesses:* Sore throat and pinkeye.

15.4 Shihhsuan

*Site:* At the tip of each finger. (Altogether there are ten points.)

76

*How to locate:* Locate the point with the patient's hand stretched. The point is at the tip of each finger, 0.1 body chun from the nail (Fig. 68).

*Associated treatment:* Penetrate with slim needle or stab this point to let blood.

*Associated illnesses:* Apoplexy or strokes (the loose type), heat-strokes, fever, cramps or spasms of the extremities. These are points for administering emergency treatment for sudden fainting.

15.5 Ssufeng

*Site:* This is a group of eight points, four on the palm of each hand, distributed on the index finger, the middle finger, the ring finger, and the little finger. Each point is centered between the upper wrinkle and the lower wrinkle of the second finger joint.

*How to locate:* Locate the points with the hand stretched, palm up (Fig. 68).

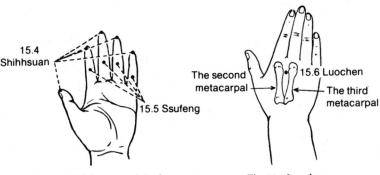

**Fig. 68**   Shihhsuan and Ssufeng          **Fig. 69**   Luochen

*Associated treatment:* Penetrate to a shallow depth, then squeeze yellowish-white transparent liquid from the needle hole on the palm side of the finger.

*Associated illness:* Swollen belly in children.

15.6 Luochen

*Site:* On the back of the hand, behind the knuckles of the index finger and the middle finger.

*How to locate:* Locate the point with the patient's hand stretched, palm down. The point is in the cavity between the second and the third finger (metacarpal) bones, above the two joints (knuckles) (Fig. 69).

*Associated treatment:* Penetrate perpendicularly to a depth of 0.1 to 0.2 chun (0.3 to 0.6 cm.). This point may also be stabbed to let blood.

*Associated illness:* Crick in the neck.

15.7 Ernih

*Site:* On the chest below the nipple.

*How to locate:* Have the patient sit upright or lie supine. The point is directly below the nipple, between the seventh and eighth ribs (Fig. 70).

*Associated treatment:* Penetrate to a depth of 0.3 chun (1.0 cm.). Moxibustion dosage is three to seven cones or five to fifteen minutes with the wicks.

*Associated illness:* Belching.

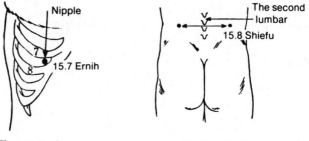

**Fig. 70**   Ernih                          **Fig. 71**   Shiefu

15.8 Shiefu

*Site:* On the back side of the waist.

*How to locate:* Have the patient assume a squatting position and lean forward. From the lower end of the fourteenth vertebra (the second lumbar vertebra), measure sideways 4.0 body chuns to either side; these are the points (Fig. 71).

*Associated treatment:* Penetrate to a depth of 3.0 chuns (9.6 cm.). Moxibustion dosage is five cones.

*Associated illness:* Failure to menstruate.

15.9 Hsiyen

*Site:* There are two points on each knee, along the baseline of the kneecap.

*How to locate:* Have the patient sit upright with his feet dangling. There are two cavities at the base of the kneecap, one on each side of the lower tip. The points are inside the cavity (Fig. 72).

*Associated treatment:* Penetrate to a depth of 0.5 chun (1.6 cm.). Moxibustion dosage is three to five cones.

*Associated illnesses:* Ache at the knee and indigestion or heartburn.

15.10 Lanwei

*Site:* On the lateral side of the lower leg.

*How to locate:* Proceed from the stomach line at 3.7 directly downward for 2.0 body chuns, then move a very small distance inward toward the center of the leg; feel for a point sensitive to finger pressure or a small solid lump. This is the point (Fig. 72).

*Associated treatment:* Penetrate perpendicularly to a depth of 1.0 to 1.5 chuns (3.2 to 4.8 cm.). Moxibustion dosage is five to ten cones or more; or wicks may be used for ten to twenty minutes.

*Associated illness:* Appendicitis.

15.11 Tiaoshan (Tiaokou–Chengshan)

*Site:* At the lower part of the leg.

*How to locate:* Seat the patient upright, with his foot dangling. First locate Tiaokou (stomach skin line) by finding the midpoint of the line joining the inner ankle tip to 11.4; then from this point move horizontally toward the front part of the leg for two index-finger widths. Tiaoshan is the tunneling line joining Tiaokou and Chengshan (7.10 on the bladder line) (Fig. 73).

*Associated treatment:* Penetrate the needle perpendicularly into the skin at Tiaokou with the tip directed toward 7.10; rotate-insert the needle until the needle tip reaches beneath the skin at 7.10. The depth of penetration should be 2.0 to 3.0 chuns (6.4 to 9.6 cm.).

*Associated illnesses:* Backache and ache at the waist.

15.12 Shiherhsing (Twelve Wells)

*Site:* This is a group of twelve points, including 1.4, 2.1, 9.4, 10.1, 5.3, and 6.1.

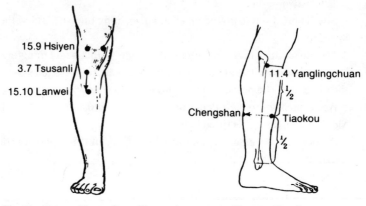

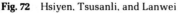

**Fig. 72** Hsiyen, Tsusanli, and Lanwei      **Fig. 73** Tiaoshan

*Associated treatment:* Penetrate perpendicularly to a depth of 0.1 chun (0.3 cm.), or stab the point to let blood.

*Associated illness:* Emergency treatment for sudden fainting and unconsciousness.

15.13 Shangpai

*Site:* Altogether there are four points: One on each thumb, at the back side of the outer edge of the thumb, near the base of the nail; one on each big toe, at the back side of the outer edge of the big toe, near the base of the nail.

*How to locate:* On the hand, the point is located at the base corner of the thumbnail (near 1.4); on the foot, it is at the base corner of the toenail (near 4.1) (Fig. 74).

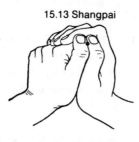

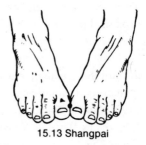

**Fig. 74** Shangpai

80

*Associated treatment:* Bind the thumbs together side by side with strips of cloth so that the two points coincide; bind the toes together in the same way. Place a cone at the point so that half the cone base is supported by the skin and the other half is on the nail. Heat three cones on the hands and three cones on the feet.

*Associated illness:* Epilepsy.


APPENDIX
# CUPPING

Cupping consists of pulling the skin by using a warm cup. The equipment is easy to set up and use. Cupping can be used very conveniently, either by itself or in conjunction with other therapy. The cupping locations on the body by and large coincide with the acupuncture points.

## 1. Types of Cups Employed

Three types of cups are commonly used. The first type is made from a bamboo segment with a small mouth and base and a slightly enlarged midsection—that is, resembling a Yao drum. The other two types are globular, small-mouthed pots made of clay and glass. The glass cup has the advantage of allowing observation of the skin surface during treatment. Each of the three types of cup is available in different sizes. Choice of size is determined by the location of the area to be treated.

## 2. Ways of Firing the Cup

a. Tossing fire: Light a wad of paper or an alcohol-soaked cotton ball and toss it into the cup. Quickly hold the mouth of the cup to the skin at the point of application. The cup will grasp the skin. Applications should be made with the cup held horizontally to avoid burning the patient.

b. Hot air: Hold the burning wad of paper or cotton ball with tweezers inside the cup for a while. Remove, and immediately apply the cup to the skin. This is one of the safest methods of cupping.

c. Swizzling with alcohol: Put a few drops of alcohol in the cup, turn the cup on its side, and roll it around until the interior of the cup is evenly covered with alcohol except for the area near the mouth. Then light the alcohol and apply the cup.

d. Fire on the side: Slightly moisten a clean cotton ball with alcohol and stick it midway down on the inside wall of the cup. Then light the cotton ball and apply the cup.

### 3. How to Apply Cupping

Cupping involves a sequence of five steps:

a. Preparation: First of all, it is necessary to set up a number of cups with various mouth sizes, a pair of tweezers, some alcohol, cotton balls, matches, soap, a towel, and a washbasin.

b. Selecting the cup: Cup size depends on the site of application. When the area of application is small or the skin is thin, as on the head or neck, use a small cup. If a large area is involved or the skin is thick, as on the hip, thigh, or back, a large cup is indicated.

c. Duration of treatment: The duration of treatment depends on a number of factors, including the sensitivity at the application site, the tightness of suction, skin thickness, and the nature of the illness. So long as the cup adheres, the skin is undamaged, and the patient is comfortable, treatment may continue. If one or more of these conditions do not hold, the duration must be lessened. When an ailment is accompanied by aches and pains, the treatment is generally longer than it would be otherwise. Longer treatments are also indicated when an illness is severe than when it is mild.

d. Removing the cup: When removing the cup, use one hand to depress the skin around the cup and the other hand to push the cup to the side so that the suction is lost along one edge of the cup's mouth. The cup will then fall away from the skin.

e. Precautions: It is normal for cupping to leave the skin moist, purplish-red, indented by the mouth of the cup, and swollen in the center. This condition will disappear in a few hours or at most in a day or two. If the color is a dark purple, a protective cotton bandage should be applied. If the skin surface is burned, medication should be applied to prevent infection. If application of a small bamboo cup has left a blister, the blister should not be cut with scissors, but rather should be popped at the base with a needle to drain and then covered with an antiseptic bandage to prevent infection.

f. Other precautions: During cupping the patient should not be allowed to catch cold. He should be kept indoors and away from drafts. It is normal for the patient to feel tightness and uncomfortable warmth at the site where the cup is being applied. If, however, the patient complains of extreme tightness or burning, the cup should be removed at once and the skin surface should be examined carefully. If there is evidence of a burn, the cup should be reapplied at a different site. If the patient appears to be overly sensitive, the treatment should be stopped. If at any time during the treatment there are indications of shock, such as dizziness, blurred vision, nausea, pallor, cold feet, cold sweats, or shortness of breath, the cup should be removed immediately and the patient should lie down. In light cases, a drink of water should suffice. In more severe situations, the methods given in Section III.10 should be applied.

### 4. Diseases Amenable to Cupping

    a. Headache, dizziness. and eye affliction from colds or flu.
    b. Common coughs, bronchial congestion, and whooping cough.
    c. Rheumatism, muscular aches and pains, leg ache, and pains around the waist.
    d. Indigestion, abdominal pain, stomachache, intestinal gas, and sudden diarrhea.
    e. Leg cramps, and vomiting and diarrhea resulting from cholera.

### 5. Conditions Where Cupping Is Forbidden

a. Cupping is forbidden at anatomical sites where there is evidence of skin disease or where the body is shriveled and there is loss of muscle tone.
b. When the patient is unconscious or having convulsions.
c. When the skin is highly sensitive or when there is swelling.
d. Near a skin tumor or a running sore or boil.

Furthermore, in pregnant women, cupping is forbidden in the abdominal area, on the breasts, and in the region near the heart.

### 6. Cupping Sites for Common Ailments

a. Colds and influenza: Cup points 15.2, 15.1, and 2.2.
b. Headache: Cup 14.6 and 15.2.
c. Whooping cough: Cup 14.4.
d. Malaria: Cup 14.6 and 14.5.
e. Skin rash: Cup 14.6, 14.3, 2.3, and 7.9.
f. Asthma: Cup 7.3, 7.4, 14.4, 13.5, and 13.3.
g. Indigestion or heartburn: Cup 13.5, 3.7, 9.3, 7.6, and 7.7.
h. Hiccups: Cup 7.3, 7.4, and 13.5.
i. Vomiting or diarrhea: Cup 3.5, 13.3, 13.2, 4.2, and 7.6.
j. Dysentery: Cup 3.5 on the *left foot,* and 13.1.
k. Abdominal pain: Cup 3.5, 13.5, and 13.3.
l. Chest pain: Cup at the site of the pain.
m. Backache at the waist: Cup 7.8 and 14.2.
n. Backache at the shoulders: Cup 14.6, 14.4, 7.3, and 7.4.
o. Aching thighs: Cup 7.8, 11.3, and 4.4.
p. Stiffness in the upper legs: Cup 11.3, 7.9, 7.8, and 3.7.
q. Inability to raise the arms: Cup 7.3, 2.4, and 2.3.
r. Aches and pains from chills, dampness, or drafts: for the arms and shoulders, cup 2.4, 2.3, 10.4, 2.2, and the site of the pain; for the legs, cup 11.3, 3.7, 11.5, and the site of the pain; for the middle back, cup 14.6, 11.3, 7.8, 14.3, and 7.9.
s. Cramps in the calf of the leg: Cup 7.10, 7.9, and 4.2.
t. Painful menstruation: Cup 13.3, 13.1, 13.2, 3.5, and 7.8.
u. White discharge from vagina: Cup 13.2, 13.3, and 4.2.
v. Redness, swelling, and pain around the eyes: Cup 15.2.
w. Waist pain from contusions: Cup 14.2, 7.8, 11.3, and 7.9.
x. Injury due to joint being twisted or from a fall: Cup the affected area.

# PART TWO

# Common Illnesses and How to Treat Them

## 1. Colds and Influenza

Colds and flu occur the year around. They usually result from sudden changes in the weather or from getting chilled after over-exertion and sweating. The symptoms are: a chilly feeling, fever, headache, cough, sneezing, runny nose, stuffy nose, aching arms and legs, general weakness, and sore throat.

*Treatment:* Locate points 14.6, 2.2, and 11.2. These three points are the principal points of treatment for colds and flu. Perform rotation-insertion with the slim hao needle, followed by a combined tone-and-tap manipulation. Leave the needle in place for a passive phase of thirty minutes. For headache, use an additional needle at 15.2; and for severe headache, add a needle at 3.4 and one at 1.2. For sore throat, use a trocar needle to let blood at 1.4. For coughing, apply a needle at either 1.1 or 7.4. For head congestion, apply a needle at 2.5. For aching in the arms, legs, and body, use needles at 2.3 and 7.10.

## 2. Cough

Coughing is a very commonly observed symptom which usually reflects illness of the lung. On the other hand, disorders of other internal organs often affect the lungs, and coughing results. Therefore, coughing is a symptom of many different illnesses. Despite this, coughing usually results from having caught a cold or from internal causes.

a. Coughing due to colds: The symptoms are chills and fever, stuffy nose, sneezing, coughing up thin and white mucus, and perhaps a headache.

*Treatment:* Locate 14.6, 11.2, 7.4, 2.2, and 1.2. These points are used with rotation-insertion of slim needles. Combine toning and tapping, and allow a twenty-minute passive phase.

b. Coughs due to internal causes: Coughing is intermittent; mucus is white and viscous if it is present at all; the throat feels hot, dry, itchy, and sore; the mouth is dry, and the lips are red. The palms of the hands and the soles of the feet may feel warm to the touch, and there may be pains in the back or chest.

*Treatment:* Locate 7.4, 7.3, 3.7, and 1.3. Tone these points with slim needles and then apply moxibustion after the needle has been extracted.

### 3. Headache

Headache is a symptom of a variety of illnesses, either contracted or from other internal causes. Here we are concerned only with illnesses in which headache is the principal symptom. Since the location of pain varies from patient to patient, the acupuncture therapy will differ accordingly.

a. *Treating a generalized headache:* There are two methods.

i. Locate 3.7, 2.2, and 11.4. Insert two slim needles into each point from opposite sides and rotate them until the patient senses soreness and numbness. Tap, using rotation. The passive phase lasts thirty minutes. The treatment should be administered once a day or once every other day.

ii. Locate 14.8, 14.10, and 10.3 and heat with three to five cones.

b. *Treatment of a headache at the top of the head:* Locate 14.8 and 1.2 and, at 14.8 on the crown, perform rotation-insertion with a slim needle at a 45-degree angle slanted toward the posterior, to a depth of 0.3 chun (1.0 cm.). At the other acupoint, 1.2, use rotation-insertion with a slim needle, to a depth at which the patient feels soreness and numbness. Follow by a thirty-minute passive phase. Acupuncture may also be administered at 11.2, 7.3, and 12.3.

c. *Treatment of pain at the temples:* There are three different treatments.

i. Locate 11.5. Rotate-insert a slim needle, tap, and leave the needle for fifteen minutes.

ii. Locate 8.1 and apply moxibustion, using three cones.

iii. Locate 3.4 and 1.2. Use a slim needle to enter 3.4 at the pain site. Insert the needle parallel to the skin and upward until a sensation of irritation occurs, and then extract it. Then insert a needle at 1.2

toward the shoulder at a 45-degree angle to the hand and leave it for thirty minutes. An additional needle may be placed at 10.7.

iv. Pain at the forehead: Treat at 14.9, 14.8, 15.2, 2.2, and 1.2.

v. Pain in the back of the head: Treat at 11.2, 10.4, 7.11, and 1.2.

vi. Pain over the eyebrows: Treat at 3.4, 7.2, 1.2, 14.10, and 10.7.

Each of these last three types of headache treatment consists of rotation-insertion of slim needles, tapping, and a passive phase of fifteen or twenty minutes.

## 4. Dizziness and Nausea

The patient complains of vertigo and blurred vision, as if he were seasick, and feels a loss of balance while standing. His vision seems to black out or spin. The condition often results from a general lack of vitality.

*Treatment:* Locate 14.8 and 8.2. First apply heat at these two points with cones. If the dizziness and nausea are accompanied by insomnia, additional moxibustion should be applied at 3.7 and 2.2. If the feeling of nausea is pronounced, use needles at 13.5 and 9.3, as well as heat at the original two points, and then apply heat to the latter two points. Finally, if the heart palpitates and the pulse is too fast, moxibustion at 14.8 and 8.2 should be supplemented by acupuncture at 5.2.

## 5. Insomnia

Insomnia is the inability to sleep sufficiently during the night. There are several different forms of insomnia. Some patients have difficulty in falling asleep. Some awake in the early dawn hours and cannot return to sleep. Others sleep so lightly the slightest disturbance will awaken them. Some insomniacs alternate sleeping and sleepless periods. Others fall asleep easily but are shortly awakened. In the most severe form, patients are unable to sleep at all for long periods. Insomniac patients often suffer from palpitations of the heart, vertigo and mild disorientation, and generalized weakness. It is often the result of anxiety.

*Treatment:* Locate 9.3, 5.2, and 4.2. Use the slim hao needle and the insertion-rotation technique. Manipulate the fingers so as to achieve a combination of toning and tapping. Then leave the needles in place for a passive phase of thirty to fifty minutes. It may help the treatment if moxibustion is applied to certain other acupoints just before the patient retires. This is done by applying moxibustion, using three cones at 4.1 and 7.12. If moxibustion given once a day for fifteen days does not relieve the insomnia, the needle treatment should be repeated.

### 6. Sunstroke or Heatstroke

Sunstroke occurs mostly during the summer, usually as a result of traveling or working outdoors for too long a time when the sun is hot. The usual symptoms are an initial suffering from headache, dizziness and nausea, weakness in the limbs, and vomiting. This is followed by sudden fainting with the teeth clenched and whiteness in the face. Severe cases may be fatal unless treated promptly.

*Treatment:* Locate 2.2, 9.3, 3.7, and 14.11. First press heavily at point 14.11 with the fingernail, and then insert slim needles at the first three points; first tap, and follow this with toning. Leave the needles in for fifteen minutes. In severe cases, additional needles may be used at 2.3 and 15.4 or, as an alternative, the trocar may be used to stab 15.12 to let blood. If convulsions occur, the trocar should be used to let blood at 7.9 and 9.1. If the heart is in discomfort or palpitates, apply an additional slim needle at 5.1.

### 7. Apoplexy or Strokes

Strokes occur mostly in older people or people who are overweight. When a stroke occurs, the victim will fall, lose consciousness, have a twisted facial expression, and suffer partial paralysis (hemiplegia). Acupuncture and moxibustion may be used to treat emergency cases. Treatment will be discussed in terms of two main categories—"tight" strokes and "loose" strokes.

a. "Tight" strokes: Following a "tight" stroke, the patient's eyes are wide open, his hands and jaw are tightly clenched, mucus in the throat makes a noise akin to that of a handsaw, the face is red, breathing is heavy, and the patient cannot urinate or have bowel movements.

*Treatment:* Locate 14.11, 15.4, 2.2, and 14.8 and use the trocar needle to stab and let blood at 14.11 and 15.4. Then use slim needles at 2.2 and 14.8, tap, and maintain a passive phase of ten to fifteen minutes. If there is excess mucus, apply additional needles at 3.8 and 1.1. If the facial expression is distorted, apply additional needles at 3.1, 3.2, and 3.3. If the patient has fever, apply additional needles at 14.6 and 2.3. If the patient's consciousness is murky, apply an additional needle at 5.2. If the arms and legs are twisted and bent, apply additional needles at 2.4 and 11.4. If hemiplegia is present, additional needles should be used at 11.3, 11.4, 11.5, and 7.9.

b. "Loose" strokes: The patient's mouth is open, eyes are closed, hands are open and relaxed, there is free urination, hands and feet are cold, the breath is shallow, and perspiration appears in beads.

*Treatment:* Locate 13.2, 13.3, 13.4, 4.2, and 14.11. Apply moxibustion with a few dozen cones at each of the first four points—13.2, 13.3, 13.4, and 4.2—applying moxibustion over salt at 13.4 on the navel. Also apply a slim hao needle at 14.11. If remission occurs, moxibustion should be administered at 14.8 and a needle used to tone at 7.8.

### 8. Epilepsy (Grand Mal)

Epilepsy usually results from conditions existing at birth or as the remnant of a childhood occurrence. On the occurrence of an attack, the patient will fall suddenly, lose consciousness, and undergo spasms in the arms and legs; his eyes will roll up and he will foam at the mouth and sometimes snort. After a while the patient usually regains consciousness and returns to normal. Attacks are irregular; they may occur only once in several years, a few times a year, or several times a month.

*Treatment:* Two methods are used.

a. Locate 15.13 on both thumbs and on the big toes, and locate 8.1. Tie the two thumbs together and the two big toes together, and heat the points 15.13 simultaneously by continuously burning several cones, at which time the patient should regain consciousness. If he remains unconscious, burn four or five cones at 8.1.

b. Locate 14.6, 14.8, 14.11, and 9.2. Apply slim needles at these points for a twenty-minute passive phase. Then remove the needles and apply moxibustion at 14.6 and 14.8. If the symptoms indicate, needles may be applied at one or more of the points Fengfu (on the back of the head at the base of the cranium), 3.2, 13.7, 5.2, 2.3, 3.8, and 6.2.

### 9. Belching

Eructation is commonly called belching. It is mainly caused by gas rushing up from the stomach, producing a burst of staccato "kuh-kuh" noises in the throat. If the symptoms occur only once or twice by accident, treatment is unnecessary. If the symptoms persist, however, the following treatment is advised:

*Treatment:* Locate 9.3. Ask the patient to inhale and have the patient extend his thumb. Insert a thin needle at 9.3 to a depth of 0.5 chun (1.6 cm.). Then have the patient exhale, and push the needle back to the 0.5 chun (1.6 cm.) depth and pull again out 0.3 chun (1.0 cm.), then inhale, push and pull, exhale, push and pull, and so on through a total of three deep breaths. Now allow a passive phase of ten to fifteen minutes. If the belching continues, apply needles at 8.2, 7.5, and 15.7.

### 10. Vomiting

Vomiting is a very common symptom of any one of a number of ailments. Often it results from infection, overindulgence in food or drink, eating something that doesn't agree with the patient, food poisoning, biliousness, or fluids blocked in the stomach. Bedside diagnoses usually fall into two categories: extreme nausea and vomiting, on the one hand, and a less violent category. The first category is characterized by immediate vomiting after eating, bad taste in the mouth, urination that is brief and turning red, and hard stools. The other type exhibits vomiting sometime after eating, desire to avoid chilling, thin bowel movements (like those of a duck), and general weakness and fatigue.

*Treatment:* Locate 2.3, 9.3, and 3.7. Insert slim needles at 2.3 and 9.3 and tap both points. Rotate-insert downward at 3.7 at a 45-degree angle to the skin, apply mixed toning and tapping, and leave the needle for a passive phase of thirty minutes. If the vomiting is of the extreme category, use additional needles at 2.2 and 3.9. If the other type is involved, apply the needles at 7.6 and 13.3, and follow by ginger moxibustion or application of hot salt over the abdominal area.

## 11. Indigestion or Heartburn

This ailment is also known as gas on the stomach and, since pain is primarily in the heart area, is often called heartburn. It may result from temperature changes, irregular eating habits, anger, or worry. It is characterized by stomach discomfort at the onset, gradually leading to indigestion, distention of the stomach, vomiting, groaning, spitting up sour fluid, stomachache either before or after meals, and loss of appetite.

*Treatment:* There are two treatments.

a. Locate 15.9 and apply a slim needle. If the case is acute, tap; otherwise tone. For an intensely ill, strong patient, first tap and then tone. For a weak patient with a light case, tone and then tap. The passive phase runs from thirty up to fifty minutes. After the needle is extracted, cover the patient with a blanket to encourage perspiring.

b. Locate 13.5, 9.3, and 3.7. Use a slim needle at each to apply push-pull tapping (light push, heavy pull), and leave the needles for thirty minutes. Repeat this treatment the following day.

## 12. Abdominal Pain

Abdominal pain is also called bellyache. It is symptomatic of various conditions, such as having a cold, losing one's temper, and hunger. The pain may manifest itself at various locations, including the entire abdominal region, or the lower abdomen, or perhaps the area around the navel.

*Treatment:* Three treatments are given.

a. Generalized abdominal pain: Locate 9.3 and 7.9. Insert a slim needle at 9.3, perform combined toning and tapping, and retain for a passive phase of five to ten minutes. Then stab 7.9 with a trocar needle to let blood.

b. Pain in the lower abdomen: Locate 4.3, and repeat the following process three times. Rotate-insert a slim needle to a depth of 0.6 chun (2.0 cm.); tap by moving the thumb back and lifting the needle halfway to the surface, and, while rotating, push back to the original depth. After this is completed, penetrate directly to a depth of 1.0 chun (3.0 cm.) and leave the needle for fifteen or twenty minutes. If the pain does not subside after this treatment, additional abdominal points, such as 13.3 and 13.2, may be treated; or, as an alternative, a slim needle may be applied at 7.7. In the absence of fever, the treatment may be supplemented with moxibustion—for example, by applying ginger moxibustion to 13.3 and 13.2.

c. Pain around the navel:.Locate 3.5 and 13.3. In the presence of fever use acupuncture only. If there is no fever, acupuncture may be followed by moxibustion at these points and, in addition, moxibustion over salt may be applied at 13.4.

### 13. Diarrhea

Diarrhea, or loose bowels, is characterized by thin, frequent bowel movements. The usual causes are careless eating—especially eating cold, raw, or contaminated foods—colds, or infection. The bedside diagnoses fall into two categories, according to whether the condition is acute or chronic. Early-morning diarrhea belongs to the latter category.

a. Acute diarrhea. Symptoms include abdominal pain, light brown and watery bowel movements which may contain mucus and undigested food particles, urination that is brief and turning red, and perhaps headache or slight fever.

*Treatment:* Locate 13.5, 3.5, and 3.7. Rotate-insert slim needles at each point, tap, and leave for a passive phase of twenty minutes. If the pain is severe, the treatment may be supplemented by moxibustion at 13.4.

b. Chronic diarrhea. In this ailment the diarrhea persists over a long period of time and occurs after meals. The patient has no appetite, has noisy intestines, a slight throbbing pain in the abdomen, and stools that consist of undigested food mixed with pussy mucus.

*Treatment:* Locate 13.5, 3.5, 7.6, 7.7, and 13.4. Apply ginger moxibustion at these points. Apply additional moxibustion at 14.3 if the stools are bloody.

c. Early-morning diarrhea. This form of chronic diarrhea is characterized by pain in the lower abdomen, followed by a single loose bowel movement which in turn leads to a cold feeling in the abdomen and the legs, sometimes accompanied by abdominal swelling.

*Treatment:* Locate 8.3, 13.3, 7.8, and 13.4. At the first three of these points, use slim needles to tone, followed by a thirty-minute passive phase. Apply further toning by rotation twice during the passive phase. This should be repeated daily or every other day. The acupuncture should be followed by moxibustion at 13.3 and 7.8, and ginger moxibustion should be applied at 13.4.

## 14. Dysentery

Dysentery usually occurs during the summer as a result of eating contaminated food or of overindulging in raw or cold foods. The principal symptom is frequent bowel movements, sometimes ten or more times in a single day. Abdominal pain occurs in waves; there is a frequent desire to move the bowels, often without results; and the bowel movements contain lumps which may be white, red, or a combination of the two. If the red predominates, the disease is called red dysentery; if there is an excess of white, it is called white dysentery.

*Treatment:* Locate 13.5, 3.5, and 3.7. Apply slim needles once a day, using rotation-insertion, a combination of toning and tapping, and a thirty-minute passive phase. If the patient has a high fever, additional needles should be applied at 14.6 and 2.3. If abdominal pain is severe, apply needles at 10.5 and 12.3. In the event of headache, apply treatment at 11.2 and 14.8. For white dysentery, apply moxibustion during the passive phase at 3.5; if the bowel protrudes, apply moxibustion at 14.8; when bowel movements are frequent and fever is absent, use moxibustion over salt at 13.4.

### 15. Cholera

Cholera is characterized by simultaneous vomiting and diarrhea. It is an acute, highly communicable disease which usually occurs during the summer or fall. Onset is sudden and results in vomiting and diarrhea, colorless urine, severe abdominal pain, greenish coloration of the lips, cold hands and feet, oily sticky perspiration, and, on occasion, stupor or cramps in the arms and legs.

*Treatment:* Locate 3.7, 13.5, 9.3, 2.2, and 3.5. Rotate-insert slim needles, use combined toning and tapping, and leave for a thirty-minute passive phase. If the patient perspires heavily and the hands and feet are extremely cold, apply moxibustion at 13.2 and 13.3. If abdominal pain persists, apply additional needles at 13.3, 4.2, and 4.3. If the patient remains in a stupor, apply needles at 10.4, 14.11, 3.10, and 12.3. If there is high fever and thirst and the patient is restless and uncomfortable, apply an additional slim needle at 7.9 and let blood at 15.4. For cramps in the calves and feet, apply additional needles at 7.11 and 7.10.

### 16. Malaria

Malaria usually occurs in the fall of the year. It is transmitted by mosquitoes. At the onset of an attack the patient undergoes severe chilling accompanied by shivering and shaking. After the chill passes, the body temperature will rise until the fever is quite high and there is profuse sweating. Attacks tend to occur in regular frequencies which may be daily, every other day, every third day, etc.

*Treatment:* Two different treatments are given.

a. Locate the *ah si* or "ouch" point one or two hours before an attack is expected. This is done by having the patient sit upright, with his clothing removed above the waist. The acupuncturist places his thumbs together, end to end and, beginning at the top of the backbone and moving downward along the spine, applies firm pressure with the balls of the thumbs about 1.5 chuns (4.8 cm.) on either side until an "ouch" point, or point of greatest sensitivity and tenderness, is located. This point is called *ah si*. Use a slim needle here to a depth of 0.3 to 0.5 chun (1.0 to 1.6 cm.) and apply moxibustion with seven cones.

b. Locate 6.2, 9.2, and 14.6. An hour or two before the attack, insert a slim needle at 14.6 in a slightly upward direction to a depth of 0.5 to 0.6 chun (1.6 to 1.9 cm.) until a feeling of numbness is felt by the patient. Then administer one or two doses of warm-needle moxibustion on this needle. Continue the treatment by applying slim needles at 6.2 and 9.2, using perpendicular rotation-insertion, combined toning and tapping, and a thirty-minute passive phase. If there is vomiting, apply additional needles at 13.5 and 9.3. For abdominal pain, use needles at 13.5 and 3.7. If there is severe headache, use needles at 14.8 and 11.2. If the patient is weak and hard lumps can be felt in the upper left quadrant of the abdomen, apply moxibustion to 7.6 and 3.7.

## 17. Constipation

Constipation is a failure to have bowel movements. Movements may fail to occur for three to five days, or sometimes even longer. When they do occur, it is only after difficulty and a great deal of straining. Constipation may be a side effect of a feverish episode, or it may result from direct causes. Therapy with acupuncture and moxibustion is most effective as a treatment for chronic constipation.

*Treatment:* Locate 10.5 and 8.3. Perform insertion by rotation at 10.5 and perpendicular insertion at 8.3. Rotate to tone and tap at both points until the points become numb and sore. Retain the needles for thirty minutes.

### 18. Bloody Stools

Bloody stools is a term referring to bleeding associated with bowel movements. The ailment appears in two different forms, prior bleeding and bleeding during and after movements. In the event of prior bleeding, the blood is usually bright red or only slightly murky. Movements are slow and uncomfortable, and the anus is swollen and sore as a result of inflammation in the lower intestine. When bleeding occurs during and after movement the blood is dark purple, there is a throbbing pain in the abdomen, there is fatigue and lassitude, and the stools are loose. This condition frequently occurs after extended illness when the patient is run down.

*Treatment:* Locate 14.3, 3.5, 14.1, 7.5, and 7.8. Burn seven cones at each of 14.3 and 7.8 and ten or more at 7.5. Then apply a slim needle at 14.1, and after penetration tilt the needle slightly upward. Following this, burn at least ten cones over this point. As a final step, burn ten or so cones at 3.5. Repeat the treatment every three days. If the anus is swollen and sore, delete the moxibustion and use the needle treatment only.

### 19. Appendicitis

Appendicitis consists of inflammation of the appendix, including the possibility of its rupture. The principal symptom is pain and sensitivity to touch in the lower right quadrant of the abdomen. The skin is tight over the area of pain; the patient has difficulty in turning over and tends to lie on his back with his right leg slightly bent. Pain intensifies whenever this leg is straightened.

*Treatment:* Locate 15.10, 13.2, and 3.7. Apply perpendicular rotation-insertion of slim needles at 15.10 and 3.7, rotate to tone and tap, and leave the needles for twenty to thirty minutes. Repeat the rotations once every five minutes during the passive phase. After the needle treatment, heat some dry salt, wrap it in cloth, place it over 13.2, and leave it for a while, replacing the salt whenever it cools off. Apply the entire treatment once or twice daily until the symptoms disappear. If the abdominal pain is severe, add a needle at 3.5, and if there is vomiting, apply a needle at 9.3; in either case, tap and leave the needles for one hour, rotating the needles once every fifteen minutes. In extremely severe cases, the treatment should be supplemented by letting blood at three points—9.1, 7.9, and 3.11.

The patient should be hospitalized if the acupuncture is ineffective or if the pain is severe.

## 20. Rheumatism

Rheumatism consists of aches, pains, and numbness in the muscles and joints. It is frequently associated with living in damp or chilly conditions. Usual symptoms include tenderness or aching and numbness in the muscles or joints of the arms and legs. In some cases the location of the pain is fixed, while in other situations the pain may be felt at various sites on the body over a period of time. The ailment is generally worse during periods of cloudy or rainy weather. At times the joints may be visibly swollen and inflamed, red, and painful, and show improvement at cool temperatures. This condition is called acute rheumatism.

*Treatment:* The location of the acupoints is dependent on the location of pain.

    a.  Pain in the shoulders: Locate 2.4, 2.3, and 10.4.
    b.  Pain in the elbows: Locate 1.1, 2.3, and 10.4.
    c.  Pain in the wrists: Locate 10.3, 1.2, 10.5, 2.2, and 10.2.
    d.  Pain in the fingers: Locate 2.2 and 6.2.
    e.  Pain in the middle back: Locate 14.4, 7.8, 7.9, and 7.11.
    f.  Pain in the hips: Locate 11.3, 7.9, and 11.4.
    g.  Pain in the knees: Locate 3.6, 15.9, 3.7, and 4.3 via 11.4.
    h.  Pain in the ankles: Locate 3.9 and 7.11.
    i.  Pain in the feet: Locate 8.2, 7.11, and 12.3.

In chronic cases, both acupuncture and moxibustion may be applied; but in cases of acute rheumatism, only the needle treatment should be used.

## 21. Backache at the Waist

Pain in the middle back often results from drafty, cold, or damp conditions or from injury due to twisting the body.

*Treatment:* Two methods of treatment are given.

a. Locate 7.8, 7.9, and 14.2. Insert slim needles at each of these points and leave for thirty minutes; if the pain is severe or the condition is of long duration, supplement the treatment with moxibustion. If the pain results from a twisting injury or bruise, let blood at 7.9. If there is also pain in the feet and legs, apply slim needles at 11.3. If the pain is extremely severe at the back of the waist, apply an additional needle at 14.11.

b. Locate 15.11 and penetrate the skin at Tiaokou (leg/normal Yang/stomach; see Fig. 73) with a long thin needle. Use rotation-insertion perpendicular to the skin and penetrate, applying rotation, until the point 7.10 has been reached at its depth beneath the skin. Then apply a combined push-pull and rotation, thus transmitting a numb, aching sensation to the waist. Leave for a ten-minute passive phase. This method of treatment is also indicated when there is pain in the shoulders.

## 22. Chest Pains

Chest pains may occur either across the front of the chest or along the rib cage, either bilaterally or on one side only. Causes include depression and worry, internal bleeding, and injury from falling.

*Treatment:* Three different methods are given.

a. Locate 9.3. Rotate-insert a slim needle; apply push-pull manipulation for three minutes and a passive phase for thirty minutes. Treatment should be repeated daily.

b. Locate 1.3 by determining the specific area that is painful under pressure. Penetrate from the perpendicular to a depth of 0.6 to 0.8 chun (1.9 to 2.6 cm.) and leave the needle for thirty minutes. Repeat daily.

c. Locate 10.5, 12.3, and 10.4. Penetrate with slim needles; apply combined toning and tapping, followed by a thirty-minute passive phase. If the pain stops, the needle should be removed. A needle at 11.6 is optional.

### 23. Bed-Wetting

Bed-wetting consists of loss of control over urination, that is, involuntary urination. There are two common varieties of this ailment. Bed-wetting, or nocturnal urination, occurs during sleep without the patient's being aware of it. It is most common in children, especially if they have been weakened by illness. The other type is characterized by either brief, frequent urination around the clock or by continuous involuntary dripping. This latter type generally occurs in elderly patients or people who have been incapacitated by illness.

*Treatment:* Locate 4.2, 12.1, 14.8, and 13.1 and apply a slim needle at each. Tone at 4.2 and 13.1 and follow with a passive phase lasting one hour. Omit the passive phase at 12.1 and 14.8. Follow the needle treatment with moxibustion at 12.1, 14.8, and 13.1.


### 24. Protruding Bowel

Protruding bowel, or rectal prolapse, is a condition in which the lower portion of the colon protrudes from the body and remains there. It frequently occurs as a result of generalized weakness, after a long spell of diarrhea or dysentery, or after extended periods of coughing. Small children and elderly people are particularly susceptible groups.

*Treatment:* Locate 14.8 and 14.1 and apply slim needles. Insert parallel to the skin at 14.8 and insert upward at a 45-degree angle at 14.1. Apply toning at 14.1 by push-pull manipulation, with greater force on the downstroke than on the upstroke. Leave the needle in for twenty to thirty minutes and then apply moxibustion. Repeat the treatment every other day.


### 25. Irregular Menstruation

Menstrual periods normally occur once every twenty-eight days, more or less. If the periods occur too early or too late, the conditions are referred to as early menstruation and late menstruation respectively. If periods are early by seven or eight days or so, or if periods occur as frequently as twice in one month, the condition is called early menstruation. If periods are delayed by as much as seven days beyond normal or occur only once every two or three months, the condition is late menstruation. Collectively, these conditions are known as irregular menstruation. This irregularity is often a result of biliousness or a generally rundown physical condition.

a. Early menstruation: Periods occur early, flow is excessive and dark red or purplish-black in color, the mouth is dry and thirsts for cold liquids, the lower abdomen is affected by pain in waves, breasts are enlarged, the patient is short-tempered and constipated, and the urine is yellowish and limited in quantity.

*Treatment:* Locate 13.3, 13.1, 4.4, 4.2, 12.3, and 7.6. Tap with a slim needle at each of these points and maintain a twenty-minute passive phase.

b. Late menstruation: Periods occur late, flow is below normal and pale in color, the patient is pallid, tires easily, is sensitive to cold, suffers dull pain in the lower abdomen, experiences dizziness and blackouts, complains of heart palpitations, and has pain at the waist.

*Treatment:* Locate 13.2, 14.3, and 7.8. Rotate-insert at each, tone, and leave for fifteen minutes. Follow this treatment with moxibustion.

### 26. Painful Menstruation

Painful menstruation refers to pain and discomfort in the female before, during, or after periods. The pain may consist of either aching or sharp pain in the abdominal area below the navel or at the waist. Usual causes include irritability or depression, exposure to cold, eating raw or cold food, and poor nutrition. Prior to or during a period, the patient will suffer sharp pains, the abdomen will be sensitive to pressure, and the breasts will be enlarged. Following the period, there will be pain in the upper abdomen which can be relieved by pressing with the palm of the hand and then lifting.

Treatment by acupuncture usually gives good results, provided it is initiated two or three days prior to the onset of pain and that it is continued over three menstrual periods.

a. Abdominal pain before and during menstruation:

*Treatment:* Locate 3.10 and 4.2. Apply thin needles, first at 3.10 and then at 4.2. Apply tapping at both points and leave the needles for twenty to thirty minutes. This treatment should relieve the pain. If, however, pain persists, apply additional needles at 2.2, 3.7, 13.2, and 13.1. One or two of these supplementary treatments should suffice in light cases, but three or four treatments are necessary when the pain is severe.

b. Postmenstrual pain:

*Treatment:* Locate 7.8, 14.3, 13.2, 3.7, and 4.2. At each of these points, use a toning method and follow up with moxibustion.

### 27. Failure to Menstruate (nonpregnant)

If a period is due and fails to occur, the condition is called failure to menstruate. The diagnosis applies to different situations. Normally a girl will begin to menstruate at about the age of fourteen. If this does not occur or if, after one or more of the periods, menstruation ceases, this constitutes failure to menstruate. Moreover, the diagnosis applies to married women who have been having regular periods but then fail to do so for several months for causes other than pregnancy, in which case other observable symptoms will also be manifested.

Poor blood, as a result of illness or of excessive bleeding in childbirth, is one cause of this condition. Symptoms include indigestion, thin or watery stools, cold hands and feet, vertigo, heart palpitations, and generalized fatigue and weakness. The condition may also result from anger or worry, eating cold food, or from exposure to cold, in which case symptoms may include discomfort or pain in the chest, pain and swelling in the abdominal area, a bitter taste in the mouth, and constipation.

a. Menstrual failure because of blood deficiency:

*Treatment:* Locate 7.8, 7.6, 13.3, and 3.7. At each point, tone, remove the needles, and apply heavy moxibustion.

b. Menstrual failure from other causes:

*Treatment:* Locate 15.8, 3.7, 4.2, and 2.2. Rotate-insert a slim needle at 15.8, tap, and retain for thirty minutes. (Do *not* rotate or move the needle during the passive phase.) Let the patient rest for about five minutes after the needle has been extracted, and then apply needles at 3.7, 4.2, and 2.2 and leave for thirty minutes. Repeat the treatment every fifth day. Other points, such as 7.5, 13.1, 12.2, 13.3, and 7.8, may also be used by treating a few of them, alternately, at each period of treatment.

### 28. Heavy Menstruation

If the vaginal flow during menstruation occurs in abnormally large amounts or seeps continuously for a long period of time, the condition is called heavy menstruation. Common causes include anger and worry, working too strenuously, and exposure to extreme changes in temperature. In everyday language the two different types of heavy menstruation are called the "avalanche" type and the "leaky roof" type. In the first type there is sudden, gushing flow; in the second, seepage over an exceptionally long period of time. Both types of ailment are usually found in women over the age of forty and are unusual in younger women.

*Treatment:* Locate 4.1 and 12.1. Apply warm-needle moxibustion at each point for twenty minutes. If heart palpitation, dizziness, or general weakness is observed. apply additional moxibustion at 14.3, 13.1, 13.2, and at 13.1.

### 29. Difficult Childbirth

Difficult childbirth consists of failure to give birth within a normal lapse of time, even though the mother has gone full term, labor has commenced, labor pains have ensued, the baby has moved to the lower abdomen, and the bag of water has broken. This condition may result from the baby being too large, the passage too narrow, the baby being improperly positioned, or from lack of vitality on the part of the mother. In the event of improper positioning of the baby or weakness of the mother, treatment by acupuncture and moxibustion is indicated.

*Treatment:* Two methods of treatment are given.

a. Use wicks to apply heat for fifteen minutes every hour for three hours, the site of application being at the outer edge of the sole of the foot immediately behind the little toe. Cones may be used as an alternative.

b. Locate 7.12, 2.2, 4.2, 12.3, and 7.11. Apply moxibustion twice at 7.12, each time for ten minutes, with a ten-minute interval between treatments. Now slowly apply rotation-insertion at 2.2, using a combined rotation and push-pull to locate the node and feel the pulling and tugging (Te Ch'i); then tone and remove the needle. In turn, insert and rotate to locate the node at 4.2, tap, and retain for half an hour. If by this time the baby has still failed to arrive, needles should be applied to 7.11 and 12.3. Tap until the mother senses numbness and swelling; leave the needles and rotate them back and forth seven times at five-minute intervals. Continue until the baby appears and birth is almost complete.

### 30. Consequences of Loss of Blood in Childbirth

Excessive loss of blood in childbirth may result in the patient's being dizzy, having blurred vision, or being unable to sit up; or, on the other hand, the patient may suffer from depression, nausea, and vomiting. In extreme cases it may be impossible to awaken the patient or open her mouth.

*Treatment:* Locate 10.5, 4.3, and 3.7 and apply slim needles. Tone at 10.5 and 4.3, and allow a thirty minute passive phase. The needle at 3.7 should then be removed and moxibustion administered at this point. If the patient is suffering from continuous cold sweats, apply moxibustion at 13.3, 13.2, and 13.4 (over salt at 13.4).

### 31. Constipation after Childbirth

Excessive bleeding, and consequent weakness, in childbirth may lead to difficulty in having bowel movements, complete absence of bowel movements for several days, or hard and dry stools. The ailment is called constipation following childbirth.

*Treatment:* Locate 10.4 and 8.3. Apply slim needles, use combined toning and tapping, and retain for thirty minutes.


### 32. Insufficient Lactation

If there is little or no mother's milk, the condition is known as insufficient lactation. It is caused by the mother being weak after childbirth and lacking in vitality.

*Treatment:* Two methods are given.

a. Locate 13.6 and apply moxibustion with a wick for twenty minutes once a day.

b. Locate 13.6 and 10.2. First, penetrate 13.6 with a large-gauge, slim needle. Penetration should be parallel to the skin and in an upward direction. Rotate the needle and move to a depth of 0.8 chun (2.6 cm.), and then reduce the depth by 0.5 chun (1.6 cm.). Now repeat the following process three times: from the present depth of 0.3 chun (1.0 cm.), return the needle upward to the depth of 0.8 chun (2.6 cm.) while performing a clockwise rotation of the needle; retreat by 0.5 chun (1.6 cm.); return the needle to the depth of 0.8 chun (2.6 cm.) with a simultaneous counterclockwise rotation; retreat by 0.5 chun (1.6 cm.). When this has been done three times, perform a counterclockwise rotation of the needle inward from the 0.3 chun (1.0 cm.) depth until the skin seems to tighten around the needle and the needle seems to be sinking. Leave the needle. Now insert another needle at 10.2. At both points the passive phase is fifteen minutes.


### 33. Baby's Lockjaw from Unhygienic Cutting of Umbilical Cord

Tetanus in a newborn baby is usually the result of applying an unsanitary procedure when cutting the umbilical cord. Symptoms are: greenish color in the lips, lockjaw (the mouth is tightly closed and the gums are clenched), refusal to nurse, possible convulsions, and arching of the back and neck. The condition usually appears four to six days after birth.

*Treatment:* Two methods are given.

a. Locate 13.4. Grind an onion into a paste, apply it to the navel, and burn cones over the paste until the odor of onion can be detected on the baby's breath. Then put a few drops of onion juice in the baby's nose.

b. Observe the greenish-blue streak going from the heart area down to the navel. Light a wick and move it to apply heat back and forth along the streak until the streak disappears.

## 34. Convulsions in Children

Convulsions in children are symptomatic of a number of illnesses and usually result from high fever. Symptoms include cramps and spasms in the arms and legs, dilation and contraction of the nostrils, and pursing of the lips.

*Treatment:* Locate 15.1, 9.4, 11.2, 7.11, 6.2, 5.2, 9.3, and also locate the root of each nail. Rotate-insert at 15.1 and at the root of each nail, using slim needles. (The root of each fingernail and each toenail in the child will be reached if the needle is applied along the nail at the center of its base to a depth of 0.1 chun [0.3 cm.].) Stab at 9.4 with a trocar needle to let blood. When there is stiffness in the back of the neck, apply a needle at 11.2. If the back and neck are arched, apply a needle at 7.11. For spasms and cramps in the arms and legs, apply a needle at 6.2. If the child cannot sleep soundly, apply needles at 9.3 and 5.2. If this treatment fails to take effect immediately, the child should be sent to the hospital for emergency treatment.

## 35. Whooping Cough

Whooping cough is a condition in which coughing comes in spells, sometimes ten or more in a single day. It is frequently a long-drawn-out illness which is sometimes called the "hundred-day cough." It is usually caused by exposure. At the onset of the illness the patient suffers from chills, fever, and nasal congestion, and there is a clear nasal discharge. Coughing becomes more severe from day to day. The patient will cough several dozen times during a single spell; double up at the waist, tongue hanging out; nose and eyes will water; and he will wheeze. The coughing spell will continue until the patient vomits or spits up mucus from the lungs, and then subside. Nosebleeds and swollen eyes may occur.

*Treatment:* Locate 1.4 and 2.1. Stab and let blood at these points every second day until the condition improves. If the patient coughs up blood with the mucus, apply slim needles to some of the points 1.1, 11.2, 14.6, 7.4, 2.2, and 2.3. It may be helpful to accompany this treatment with cupping at 14.4.

### 36. Diarrhea in Children

This condition usually occurs during the summer as a result of overeating, eating contaminated food, drinking too much cold water, eating cold or raw food, or overexposure to heat or direct sun. In addition to having frequent, thin bowel movements, the child may also vomit, have pain in the abdomen, or have noise in the intestines.

*Treatment:* Locate 14.8 and slowly insert a slim needle downward along the scalp to a depth of 0.1 to 0.2 chun (0.3 to 0.6 cm.). Retain for one hour. During the passive phase, stroke the hands and fingers as follows: firmly massage from 2.1 down the index finger to the web between the thumb and index finger; repeat thirty times. Now massage the thumb eighteen times, moving from the inner side of the base of the nail down to the same web. Finally massage seven times along the path from 1.3 downward to 5.2, first moving along the thumb and heel of the hand to the center wrist and then along the wrist wrinkle.

### 37. Swollen Belly in Children

Distention of the abdomen in children is usually a result of malnutrition. The child will be emaciated, belly swollen, veins enlarged. He will throw up his milk, his stools will have an unpleasant, sour odor, and the urine will be cloudy. Crying will fail to produce tears, appetite will be poor, the skin will appear rough, there will be dry scalp and loss of hair, the face will be pallid, and the temperature will be elevated at night.

Treatment: Locate 15.5 at each one of its eight sites. Stab each of these points with the trocar needle and squeeze out the white fluid at each point until blood appears. Repeat the treatment every four days. If the child has diarrhea, apply a slim needle at each of 13.5, 3.5, and 3.7 by inserting, rotating a few times, and extracting.

## 38. Mumps

Mumps is a contagious disease which usually occurs during the winter or spring. It tends to commence in the stomach and settle in the parotid glands. It usually occurs in children between the ages of four and fifteen and is much more serious when contracted by adults. Swelling may occur on one or both sides of the neck and, in severe cases, these locations may appear red and inflamed. Pain is severe and intensifies during jaw movement, as when eating. The condition normally subsides after six or seven days.

Treatment: Locate 11.2, 10.6, 3.2, 2.2, 10.4, and 2.3. At each point rotate-insert, tap, and leave for fifteen minutes. Repeat the treatment daily.

## 39. Boils or Red Streaks

Boils are a rather common skin disorder. They are frequently observed on the head, face, arms, and legs. The center of the boil usually has a small head and a distinct core, thus having the appearance of a small nail driven into the surface of the skin. Initially there is a whitish head resembling a small grain of rice, a yellow blister, or a small purplish-black center. The surrounding area is swollen and painful, inflamed, sensitive to cold, and red in color. In light cases, the head of the boil will eventually rupture and the pus will drain out. At this point the swelling will vanish and the pain will cease. In severe cases, the area around the boil will become numb and the head of the boil will collapse and turn gray. When this happens, the poison will be absorbed into the body and the patient's life may be endangered. There is also a related condition that consists of a red, threadlike streak on an arm or leg.

*Treatment:* Locate 14.4; 2.2, and 7.9. Stab 14.4 to let a small amount of blood and immediately cup for ten minutes. If the boil is on the face, apply the needle at 2.2; if it is on the back, apply a needle at 7.9. To treat a red streak on an arm or leg, use the trocar needle to lift and cut the streak, thus draining out the poisonous blood. Begin by lancing at the point of infection and repeat every 2 or 3 chuns (6.4 or 9.6 cm.) until the end of the red streak has been reached.

## 40. Skin Rash

Skin rashes tend to appear and disappear sporadically. Individual eruptions vary in color and range from tiny pimples up to lumps the size of a pea. They may occur in flat patches, or the involved area may be swollen. The condition usually worsens after exposure to the wind. At the onset the skin is itchy. Swelling and inflammation develop when the area is scratched, and the scratching leads to intensified itching. The itching is especially severe at night.

*Treatment:* Two methods are applied.

a. Locate 6.2 and use a slim needle to penetrate in the direction of the center of the palm, rotating very slowly until the depth is 0.8 chun (2.6 cm.) and the patient reports a sensation of aching and numbness. Maintain a passive phase lasting from thirty to fifty minutes. Repeat every two days.

b. Locate 2.3, 4.4, and 7.9, and rotate-insert slim needles at 2.3 and 4.4; leave for thirty minutes, and rotate slowly during extraction. Use the trocar needle to let blood at 7.9. If the rash exudes a yellow discharge, the needle treatment should be supplemented with moxibustion at 2.3. If there is pain in the abdomen, apply needles at 13.3 and 13.5.

## 41. Crick in the Neck

A crick in the neck usually results from sleeping on a pillow that is too high or hard or from sleeping in a draft. When the patient awakens, his neck will be stiff, his head bent to one side, and he will have difficulty turning his head.

*Treatment:* Locate 15.6 and 11.5. Tap at 15.6 and apply a push-pull at 11.5 to achieve combined toning and tapping (do not rotate). Apply the treatment at 11.5 on both ankles simultaneously, and allow a passive phase of twenty minutes. Additional needles may also be applied at 6.2 and 14.6.

## 42. Pulled Muscle

Pulled muscles may result from heavy labor, athletics, lifting heavy objects, or an accidental fall. Injury is usually near a joint. The affected area may be either red and inflamed or appear black and blue. This discoloration will be accompanied by aches and pains.

*Treatment:* Locate the *ah si,* or "ouch" point. Insert needles both at this point and at the pain site, and retain them for ten minutes, at which time the patient should sense relief. If the injury is of recent occurrence, omit the passive phase and remove the needles as soon as Ch'i has been struck. In an old injury, the passive phase may be supplemented with moxibustion after the needle has been removed.

## 43. Deafness

Muteness is frequently the result of deafness. The condition may exist from birth or it may result from later damage. If a baby is born deaf, he may never learn to talk. Subsequent occurrence of deafness often follows periods of high fever. The first type cannot be very effectively treated by acupuncture, but the postfever deafness usually responds after a short period of treatment.

*Treatment:* Locate 11.1, 6.3, 10.6, 10.4, 14.7, 2.2, and 14.8. Rotate-insert at each of these points, and also rotate the needles at the time of their extraction. Each point should be tapped and given a thirty-minute passive phase. Treatment should be repeated every second day for sixty days. If there is no improvement at the end of this period, treatment should be continued for an additional sixty days.

### 44. Nosebleed

Though nosebleeds may result from injury, they usually occur spontaneously from internal causes. Frequent nosebleeds may cause blurred vision, tinnitus, pallor, and general weakness.

*Treatment:* Locate 1.4 and 14.8. First let blood at 1.4, and then use a wick to apply heat at 14.8 for ten minutes; alternatively, burn seven cones at 14.9.

### 45. Sinus Trouble

Sinus trouble usually results from one or more internal disorders. It is characterized by frequent discharge of yellowish, ill-smelling mucus from the nose, sometimes accompanied by coughing and mild headaches.

*Treatment:* Locate 2.5. First apply slim needles slightly below the inside corner of each eye, inserting downward along the skin to a depth of 0.5 chun (1.6 cm.). Then apply needles at 2.5 at a 45-degree angle to the skin and upward to a depth of 0.5 chun (1.6 cm.). Tap and leave for twenty minutes. An additional needle may be used to tap at 2.2. The treatment should be repeated every second day until the patient is relieved.

### 46. Sore Throat

Sore throat frequently results from a cold, flu, or other upper-respiratory disorder. It is usually accompanied by fever, often low grade but sometimes high. Sometimes a sore throat may precede the onset of a fever and vanish as the fever rises. Sore throats usually respond well to acupuncture and moxibustion therapy.

*Treatment:* Locate 2.2, 1.4, and 15.3. Rotate-insert at a 45-degree angle, needle tip upward, at 2.2, using a vigorous rotation; apply combined toning and tapping, and retain for twenty minutes. Now stab with a trocar needle to let blood at 1.4 and 15.3. Additional needles may be applied at 12.3 and 3.10.

## 47. Toothache

Toothache is a very common ailment which may result from an internal disorder or from a more direct cause, such as a cavity. Acupuncture and moxibustion therapy is very effective on toothache when it is related to internal disorders; relief from pain is often immediate.

*Treatment:* Three methods are suggested.

a. Locate 7.3 and apply a slim needle. Rotate in very slowly. If the toothache is on the right side of the mouth, use 7.3 on the right side of the spine; if pain is on the left, apply the needle to 7.3 on the left side of the spine. After the node is felt (Te Ch'i), leave the needle for thirty minutes.

b. Locate 12.2 and rotate-insert a slim needle in the direction of the heel to a depth of 1.0 chun (3.2 cm.).

c. Locate 3.2 and 2.2. First apply a slim needle to 2.2, with the point of the needle aimed toward the arm. Rotate strongly until the patient's aching, puffy sensation reaches the head. Then lift the needle back to skin depth, and redirect toward the index finger until the sensation reaches the fingertips. Now repeat this entire maneuver two more times. Treatment at 3.2 then follows in the form of combined toning and tapping, plus a twenty- to thirty-minute passive phase; repeat this daily. If the pain is in an upper tooth, apply additional needles at 3.10 and 3.3; if a lower tooth is involved, apply the needles at 1.2, 3.7, and 3.10. When the pain is in a gum, apply needles at 2.3 and 3.7. If the patient has a cold or fever, use needles at 14.6 and 10.4. All of the supplementary procedures require tapping at the indicated points.

## 48. Pinkeye

Pinkeye is an acute, highly contagious eye disease. Symptoms include sudden redness, swelling, and soreness on the whites of the eyes; sensitivity to light; the eyes water; a yellow, sticky substance appears around the eyes and may result in the lids being adhered

113

after a night's sleep; redness and swelling occur beneath the eye in severe cases.

*Treatment:* Three methods are given.

a. Locate 14.6 and use the trocar needle to form a horizontal row of needle holes extending 0.5 chun (1.6 cm.) to either side of 14.6. The stabs should be just sufficient to bring a drop of blood. Now cup this area for ten minutes or so.

b. Use a trocar needle to stab the small purple vein behind each ear, and let blood.

c. Locate 2.2, 1.4, and 2.1. Rotate-insert a slim needle at 2.2, and leave for ten minutes. Now bleed 1.4 and 2.1. A needle at 12.3 is optional.

### 49. Windburned Eyes

Windburned eyes refers to an eye condition in which the eyes water as a result of exposure to the wind. The condition is usually more severe in the winter than in the summer, though this is not necessarily true of chronic cases. In a severe case, there may be lesions on the eyelids, impaired vision, and occasional headaches and dizziness.

*Treatment:* Locate 11.2. At 11.2 on the left side, insert in the direction of the right eye socket, and at 11.2 on the right, aim toward the left socket, using slim needles in both cases. Maintain a passive phase for one hour. If there is continuous watering of the eye, apply additional needles at 7.2, 7.1, and 2.5.

# Numerical Listing
# of Acupuncture Points

1. **Arm/Most Yin/Lung**
   - 1.1 Chihtse
   - 1.2 Liehchueh
   - 1.3 Yuchi
   - 1.4 Shaoshang
2. **Arm/Normal Yang/Colon**
   - 2.1 Shangyang
   - 2.2 Hoku
   - 2.3 Chuchih
   - 2.4 Chienyu
   - 2.5 Yinghsian
3. **Leg/Normal Yang/Stomach**
   - 3.1 Titsang
   - 3.2 Chiache
   - 3.3 Hsiakuan
   - 3.4 Touwei
   - 3.5 Tienshu
   - 3.6 Tupi
   - 3.7 Tsusanli
   - 3.8 Fenglung
   - 3.9 Chiehhsi
   - 3.10 Neiting
   - 3.11 Litui
4. **Leg/Most Yin/Spleen**
   - 4.1 Yinpai
   - 4.2 Sanyinchiao
   - 4.3 Yinlingchuan
   - 4.4 Hsuehhai
5. **Arm/Least Yin/Heart**
   - 5.1 Tungli
   - 5.2 Shenmen
   - 5.3 Shaochung
6. **Arm/Most Yang/Small Intestine**
   - 6.1 Shaotse
   - 6.2 Houshi
   - 6.3 Tingkung

7. **Leg/Most Yang/Urinary Bladder**
   - 7.1 Chingming
   - 7.2 Tsanchu
   - 7.3 Tachu
   - 7.4 Feishu
   - 7.5 Keshu
   - 7.6 Pishu
   - 7.7 Weishu
   - 7.8 Shenshu
   - 7.9 Weichung
   - 7.10 Chengshan
   - 7.11 Kunlun
   - 7.12 Chihyin
8. **Leg/Least Yin/Kidney**
   - 8.1 Yungchuan
   - 8.2 Taihsi
   - 8.3 Chaohai
9. **Arm/Normal Yin/Pericardium**
   - 9.1 Chutse
   - 9.2 Chienshih
   - 9.3 Neikuan
   - 9.4 Chungchung
10. **Arm/Least Yang/Triple Warmer**
    - 10.1 Kuanchung
    - 10.2 Yemen
    - 10.3 Yangchih
    - 10.4 Waikuan
    - 10.5 Chihkou
    - 10.6 Yifeng
    - 10.7 Ssuchukung
11. **Leg/Least Yang/Gallbladder**
    - 11.1 Tinghui
    - 11.2 Fengchih
    - 11.3 Hsuantiao
    - 11.4 Yanglingchuan

# Alphabetical Listing of Acupuncture Points